WHITEBOARD

SAFETY

Updated

Anthony Thomas Hincks

Copyright © 2012 Anthony Thomas Hincks

All rights reserved.

ISBN-13: 978-0980873511 (Anthony Thomas Hincks)
ISBN-10: 0980873517

DEDICATION

I would like to dedicate this book to the following people:-

My wife who has been there with me over the years and has given me all of her support;

Glenn at OH & S who gave me the encouragement to go ahead with my dreams and achieve my goals;

Rob, Bronwyn and Carol also at OH & S who also gave me support;

Erik, Robyn & the guys who started all of this madness off with their cartoon adaptations of the people that worked there;

Graeme the mine general manager who at the time could see that my idea had merit and did not discourage me from continuing with it;

Tony who hired me the first time and gave me my start within the mining industry;

Family & friends who we have left behind and to the new one's that we have met.

And finally I would like to dedicate this book to all of those people that practice 'safeticality' and to those that need to learn that there are others out there who want to go home at the end of the shift, just as much as they do.

Thank you

Anthony Thomas Hincks

EVERYBODY DESERVES THE RIGHT TO BE SAFE

INTRODUCTION

'Whiteboard Safety' is another safety tool that anybody can use. It doesn't depend on what graduate studies you have done. Just as it does not depend on your drawing abilities or your poetic assumptions on life and its influences and it is meant to be fun and an interactive way of seeing safety.

Not only used within the work industry, but it can also be used by teaching institutions to introduce safety ideas on all ages.

This book was written mainly for the mining industry but it can be utilized by many work places or schools.

That is the beauty of 'Whiteboard Safety' it can be done anywhere where a whiteboard, blackboard or any other writing medium is present.

It does not depend on 'Political Correctness' because that does not save people's lives; PEOPLE DO, but in saying that, we need to be careful that it does not creep over into what is called Discrimination.

Also words may be 'Mispelled' for spelling does not save people's lives; PEOPLE DO, but spelling can be used as a tool, which is something to use and not depend on.

Drawing a picture that is perfect or in the realm of Leonardo Da Vinci is not a requirement, a person could draw stick figures and still get the point across, so drawing does not save a person's life; PEOPLE DO.

So you see, anyone or a person of any age can use this and develop it as they see fit, because Whiteboard Safety is just a safety that all people can use.

THINK SAFE - BE SAFE - STAY SAFE

WHAT STARTED THIS WHITEBOARD SAFETY METHOD

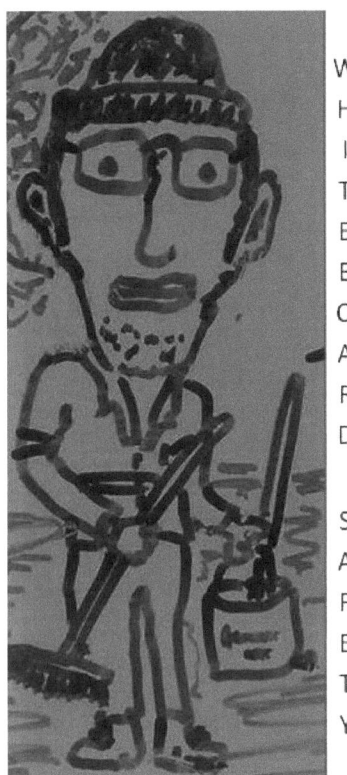

Let me introduce myself. My name is Anthony Thomas Hincks and I used to work as an Industrial Night Cleaner at a goldmine in Western Australia.

It's not some people's idea of a rewarding job, but then "what would be everyone's idea of the perfect job?" I have done a variety of jobs in the past and each time you learn different aspects of life and put them to good use.

I mean; "that's what life is all about".

One of the contractors that came to site had some drawings up on a whiteboard, of the people that worked there and because 'I felt' that I did too; I drew a picture of myself; Crazy, but true.

Not long after that I drew my first 'safety' picture which was of a dozer going through a fence because his brakes had failed. I then drew some more, on different occasions and had different themes for each of those.

To those of you reading this, the drawings only took from 2 - 3 minutes to draw from their inception to the finished product.

Using my mobile phone, cause I love to hear from my wife, I took a picture of each of them so that I would have a record of them.

One afternoon when I was showing some-one around so that they could do my job, while I had a break, I went down to the offices where I was drawing these 'safety' pictures and the guys there were having their afternoon break.

They "thanked" me for the drawings and asked if my 'replacement' would be drawing the same type of stuff, I said "No" and they were disappointed.

It seems that they would come in and hold their morning meetings where the pictures were on the whiteboard and then they would discuss the different aspects of what I had drawn or said. They even started to leave their own drawings, so that I could share in their safety thought processes.

I have been a Safety Rep before and have even written a short safety course, so I guess SAFETY is always there with me and always will be.

Just as I know this will be not everyone's 'cup of tea', what matters is that this can be used as just another tool, light hearted as it may be, but a tool none the less that anyone can utilize, at any time of the day or night.

Well, that's me and what started all of this, so short of telling you my life's story, which would take too long, I believe that we are all here for the same reason.

We want to be safe at work, at home and we want those around us to be safe as well, because life is too short to waste on not doing something safe and having no life at all.

PSYCHOLOGY OF THE DRAWINGS

When I draw the different cartoons and add the sayings, I try to gauge the 'mood' or the 'psychology' of the people in the area that I am targeting.

When I started doing the Whiteboard Safety in the mining department, I started to use fairly serious sayings combined with the cartoons.

The reason for this was because I believed that they would be better received if they were more deliberate in their concept.

It wasn't until the 4th or 5th drawing that I was a little bit more humorous in the cartoon drawings.

The reverse may also be true for a workshop Environment. You may go for the funny side first and then 'chuck' in a curve ball, by having a serious safety topic in mind.

Whichever way you go, there is no right or wrong way, but only trial and error. If they don't like one approach, then it's only reasonable to try a different one next time. Never be put off by negative comments because no matter what is said, SAFETY is and should be everyone's concern.

REMEMBER

SAFETY STARTS WITH YOU

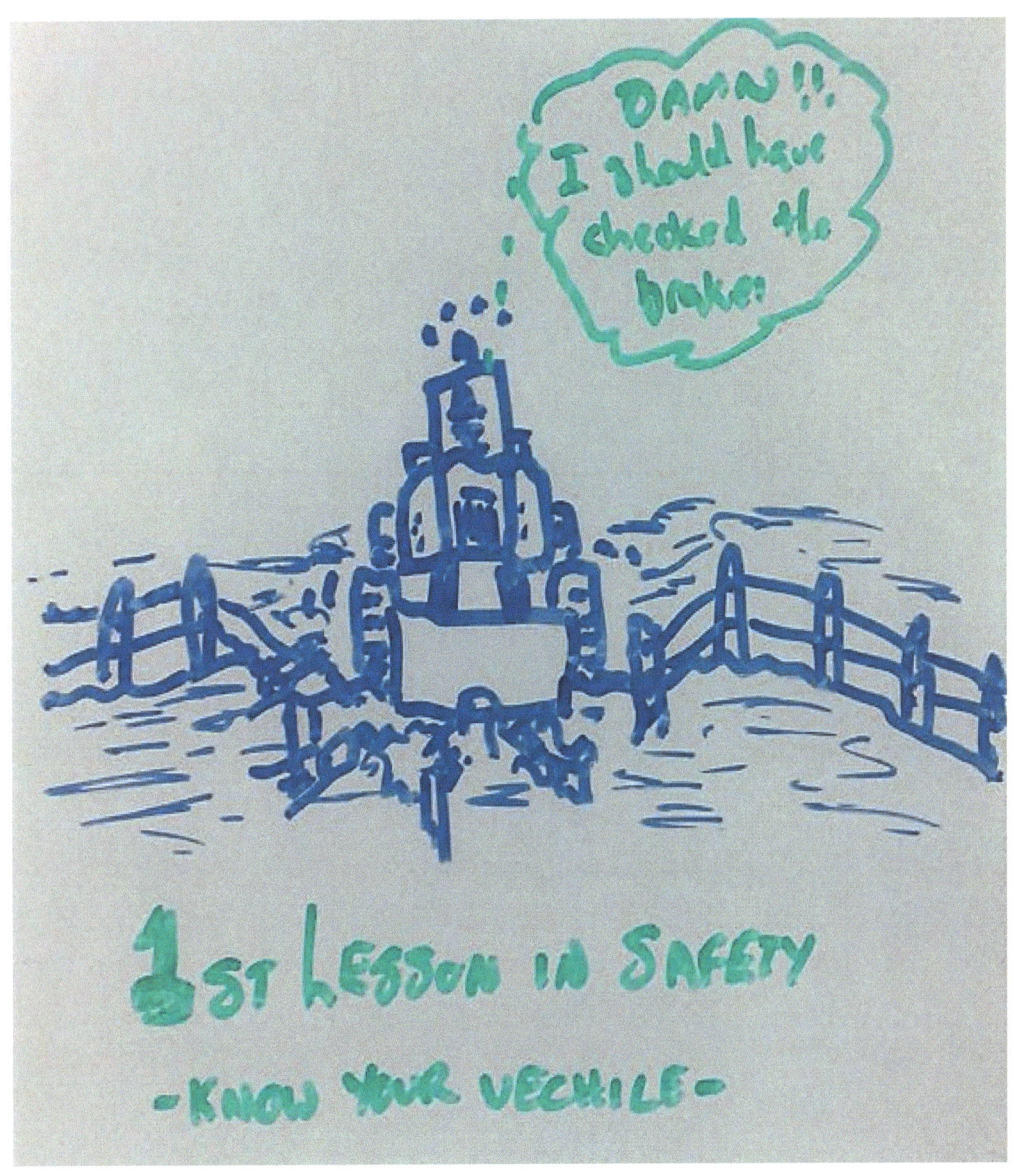

THE LESSON HERE IS THAT EVERYONE SHOULD CHECK THE VEHICLE THAT THEY ARE DRIVING BEFORE THEY START.

THIS IS CALLED 'DOING A PRESTART' AND THIS CAN BE DONE EITHER AT HOME OR WORK. THE CHOICE IS YOURS TO MAKE.

REMEMBER THAT YOU ARE IN CHARGE OF WHATEVER VEHICLE YOU DRIVE.

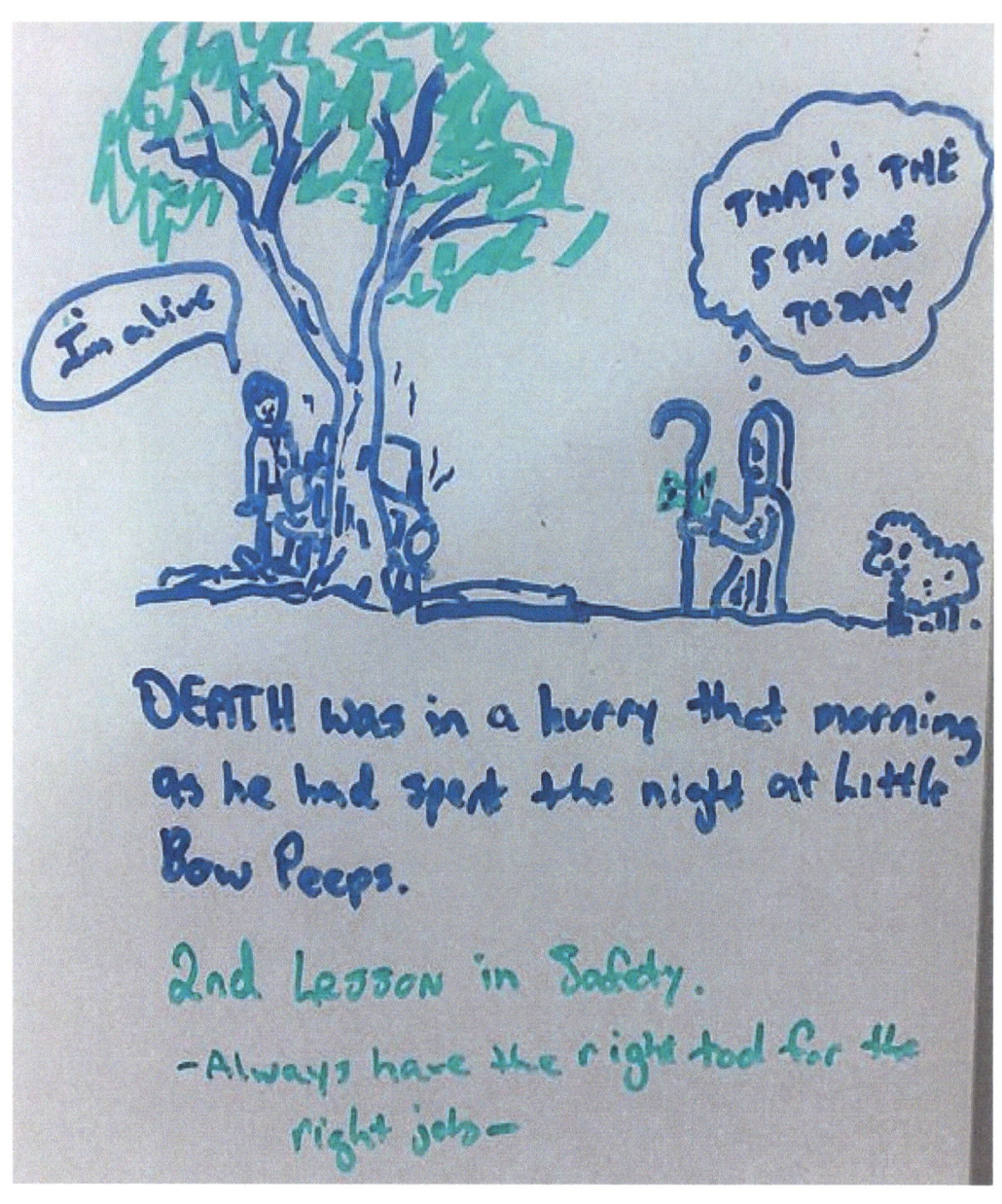

HERE WE LEARN THAT HAVING THE RIGHT TOOL FOR THE RIGHT JOB MEANS THAT WHEN YOU START ANY TYPE OF JOB OR WORK; YOU HAVE THE RIGHT TOOLS TO COMPLETE THE TASK AT HAND.

IF YOU DON'T, WELL YOU MAY TAKE LONGER THAN YOU EXPECTED TO COMPLETE THE TASK AT HAND.

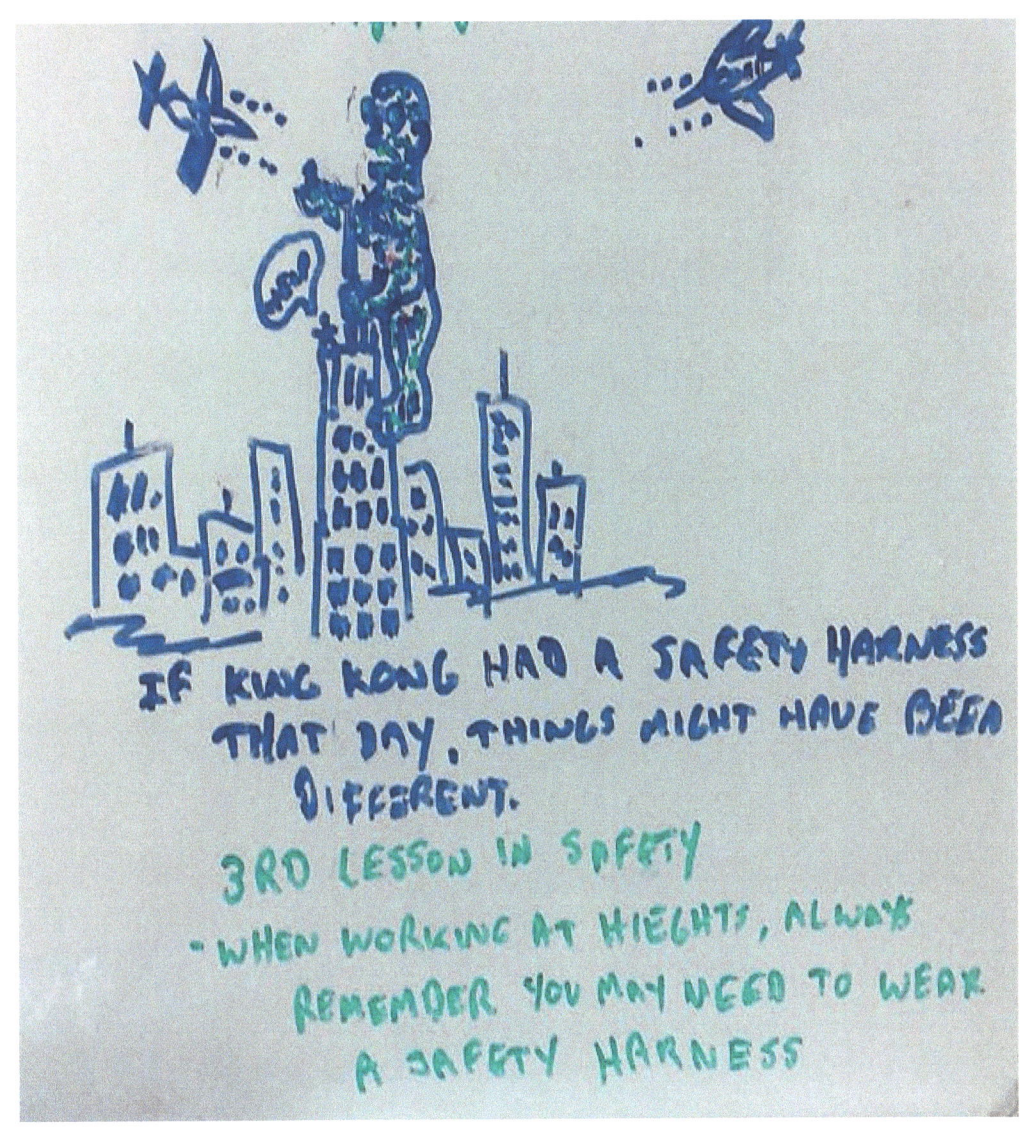

WORKING AT HEIGHTS IS DANGEROUS AND CAN HAVE DIRE CONSEQUENCES.

NORMALLY YOU WOULD NEED TO WEAR SAFETY HARNESS IF YOU ARE WORKING OVER A CERTAIN HEIGHT OR AT LEAST HAVE ANOTHER PERSON HELP YOU OR WEAR A DIFFERENT SAFETY HARNESS.

SOMETIMES EVEN A SMALL FALL CAN RESULT IN A SERIOUS INJURY.

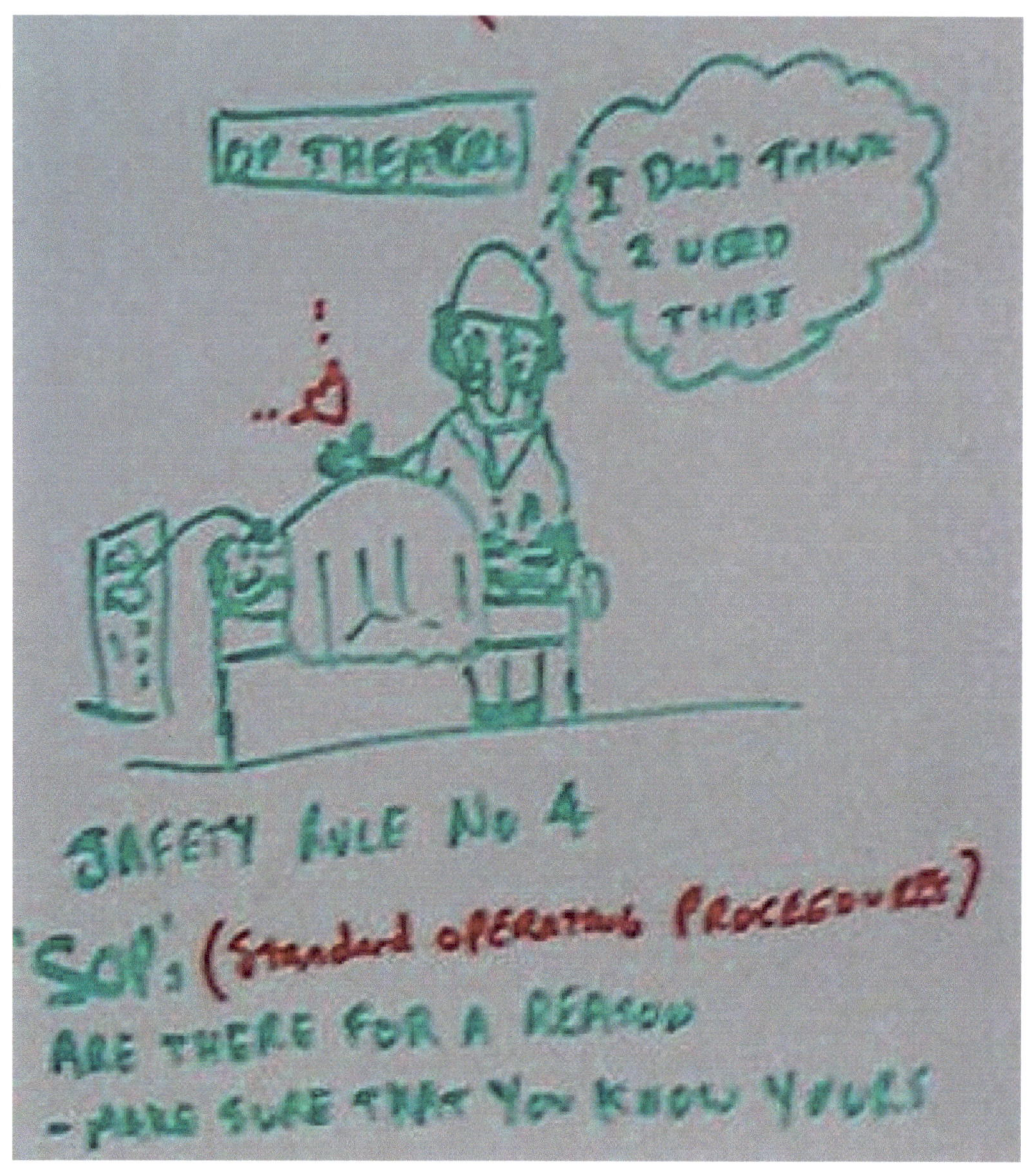

'SOP'S OR STANDARD OPERATING PROCEDURES'

THOSE LOVELY LITTLE RULES THAT WE ALL HAVE TO LIVE BY WHEN WE ARE IN THE WORKPLACE.

YOU CAN EITHER 'LOVE' THEM OR 'HATE' THEM, BUT THE REASON THEY ARE THERE IS TO PROTECT YOU FROM ANYTHING DANGEROUS FROM HAPPENING AND TO MAKE SURE EVERYTHING IS DONE IN A SAFE & PROFESSIONAL MANNER.

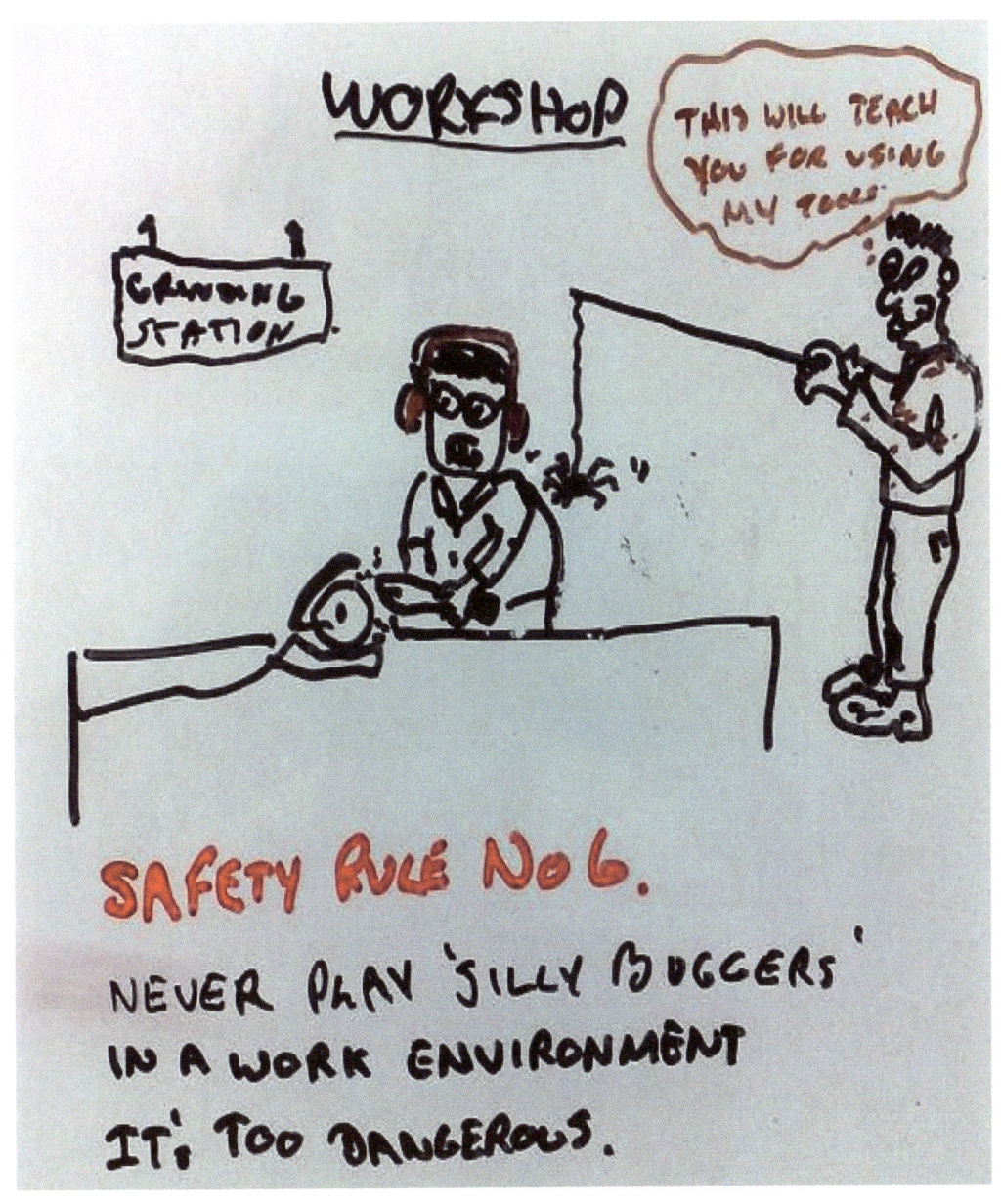

ANY TYPE OF 'SILLY BUGGERS' OR 'TOM FOOLERY' AT WORK CAN AND WILL MOST LIKELY HAVE DISASTROUS CONSEQUENCES.

MANY TIMES WE DO SOMETHING STUPID OR WITHOUT THINKING. ALL OF US HAVE BEEN GUILTY OF THIS AT ONE TIME OR ANOTHER, ME INCLUDED; BUT WHEN WE DO THIS IN A WORK ENVIRONMENT THEN WE CAN CAUSE ACCIDENTS, WHICH CAN AFFECT EVERYONE'S LIVES.

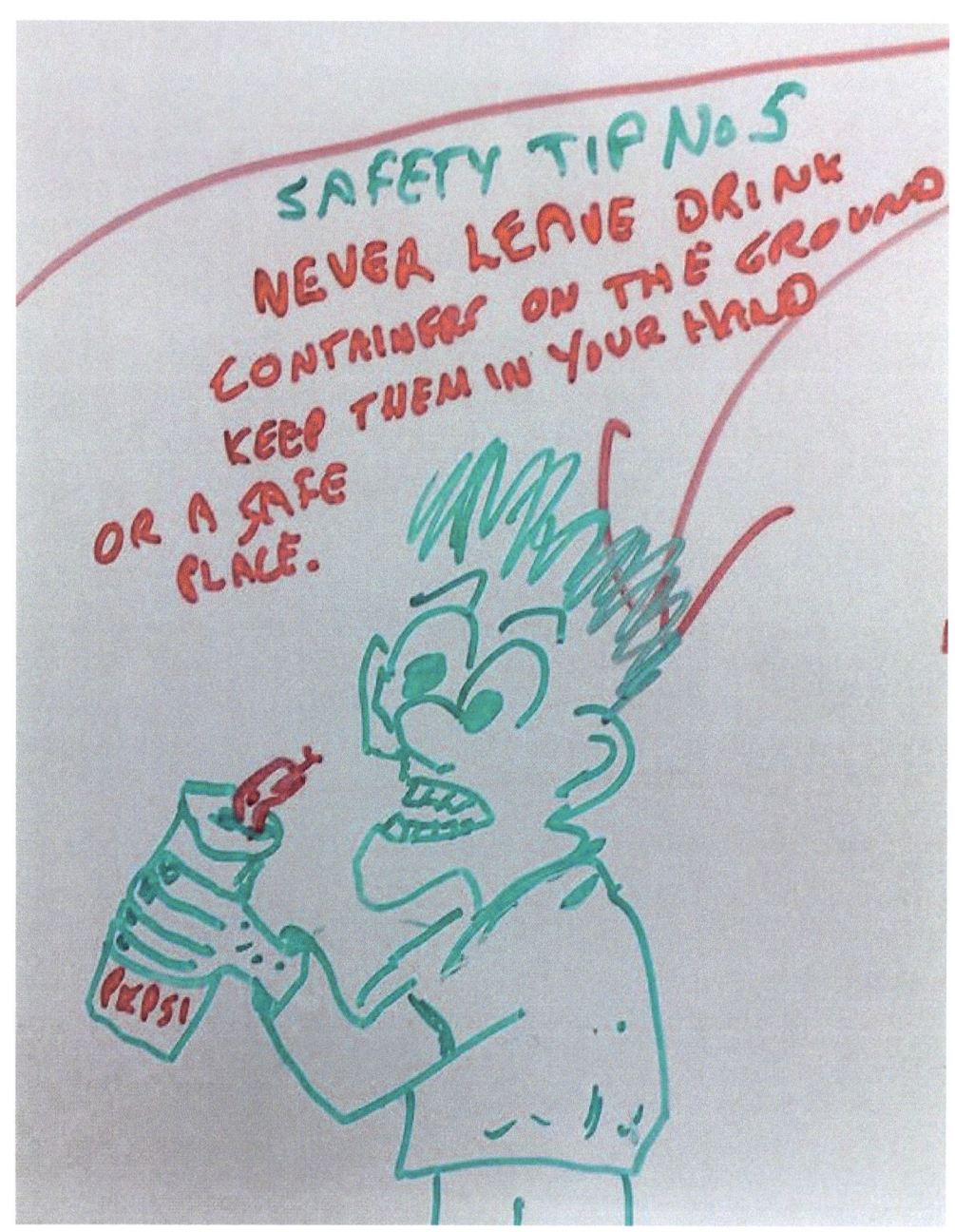

EVEN AS CHILDREN WE WERE TOLD "NEVER TO LEAVE DRINK CONTAINERS ON THE GROUND", BUT I FEAR THAT SOME OF THESE LESSONS LEARNED AS A CHILD HAVE GONE UNHEEDED.

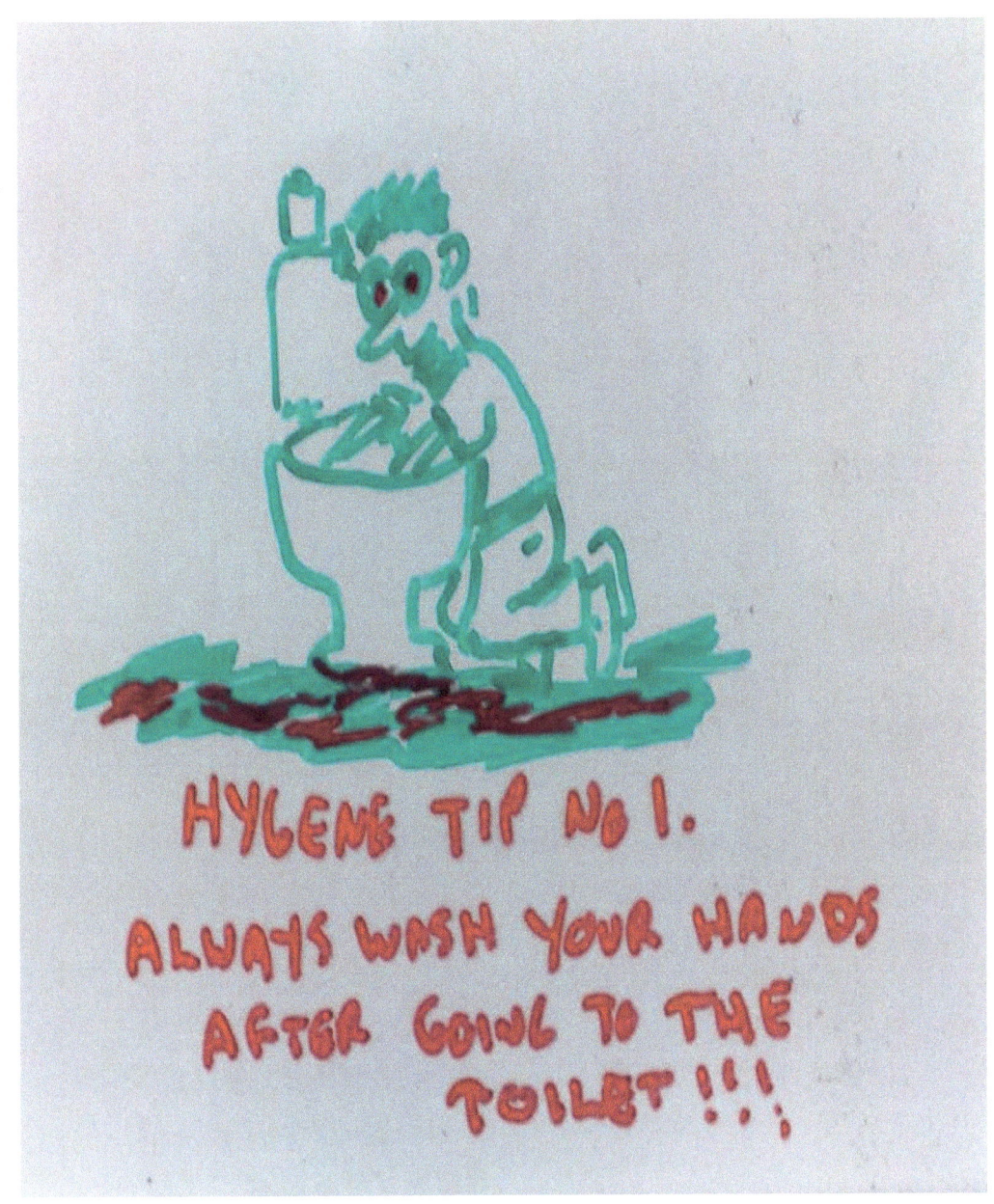

"ALWAYS WASH YOUR HANDS."

HOW MANY TIMES HAVE WE HEARD THAT FROM OUR PARENTS AND MANY, MANY OTHERS?

WE ALL KNOW THAT AFTER YOU GO TO THE TOILET THAT YOU SHOULD ALWAYS WASH, TO STOP THE SPREAD OF GERMS, BUT SOMEHOW, I DON'T THINK THEY MEANT IT QUITE LIKE THIS.

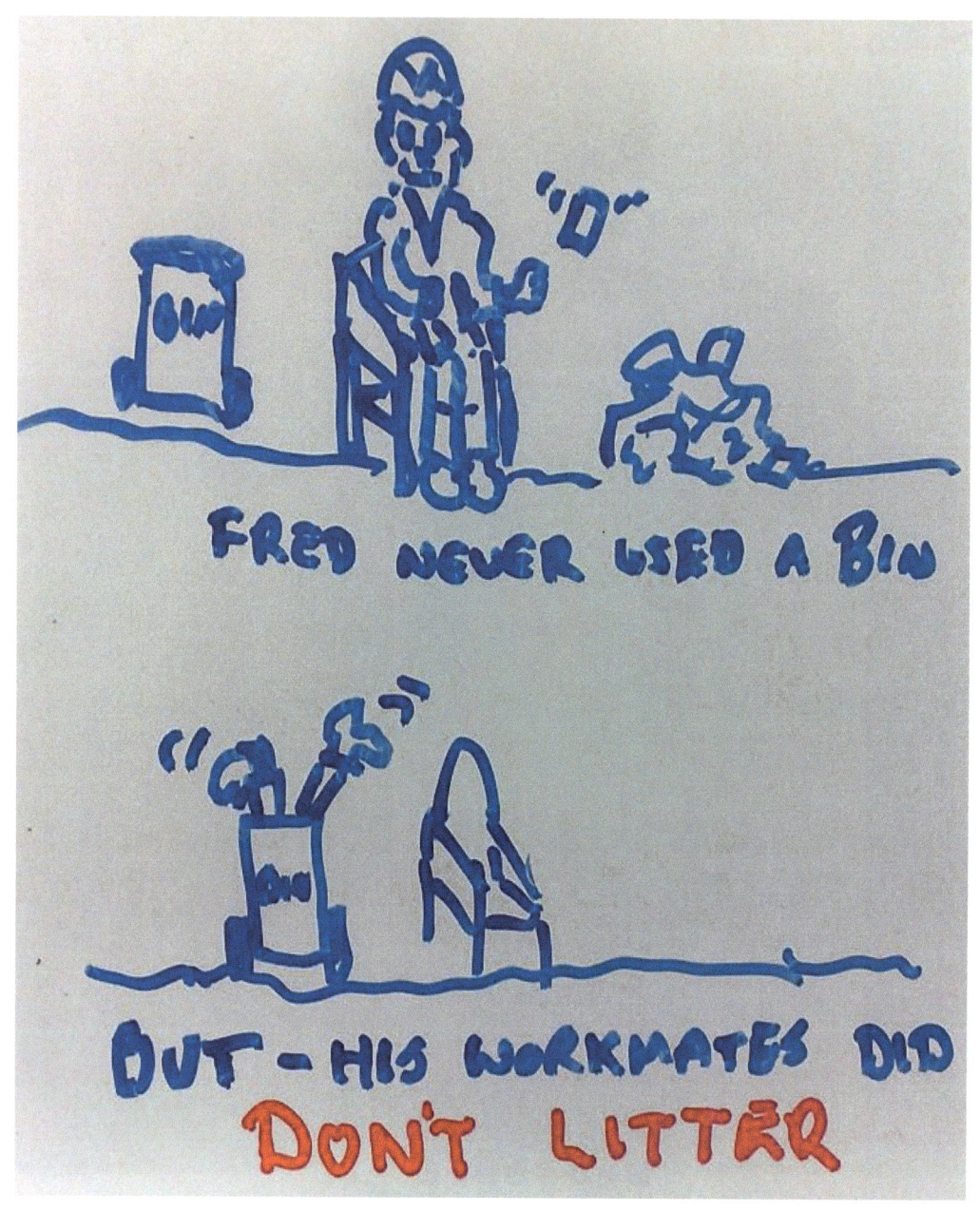

"LITTER…LITTER…LITTER"

WHAT CAN I SAY, EXCEPT THAT WE SHOULD ALL TAKE CARE WITH OUR WASTES.

THE ENVIRONMENT IS A SPECIAL PLACE AND THE MORE WE POLLUTE IT, THE SMALLER & LESS BEAUTIFUL IT BECOMES.

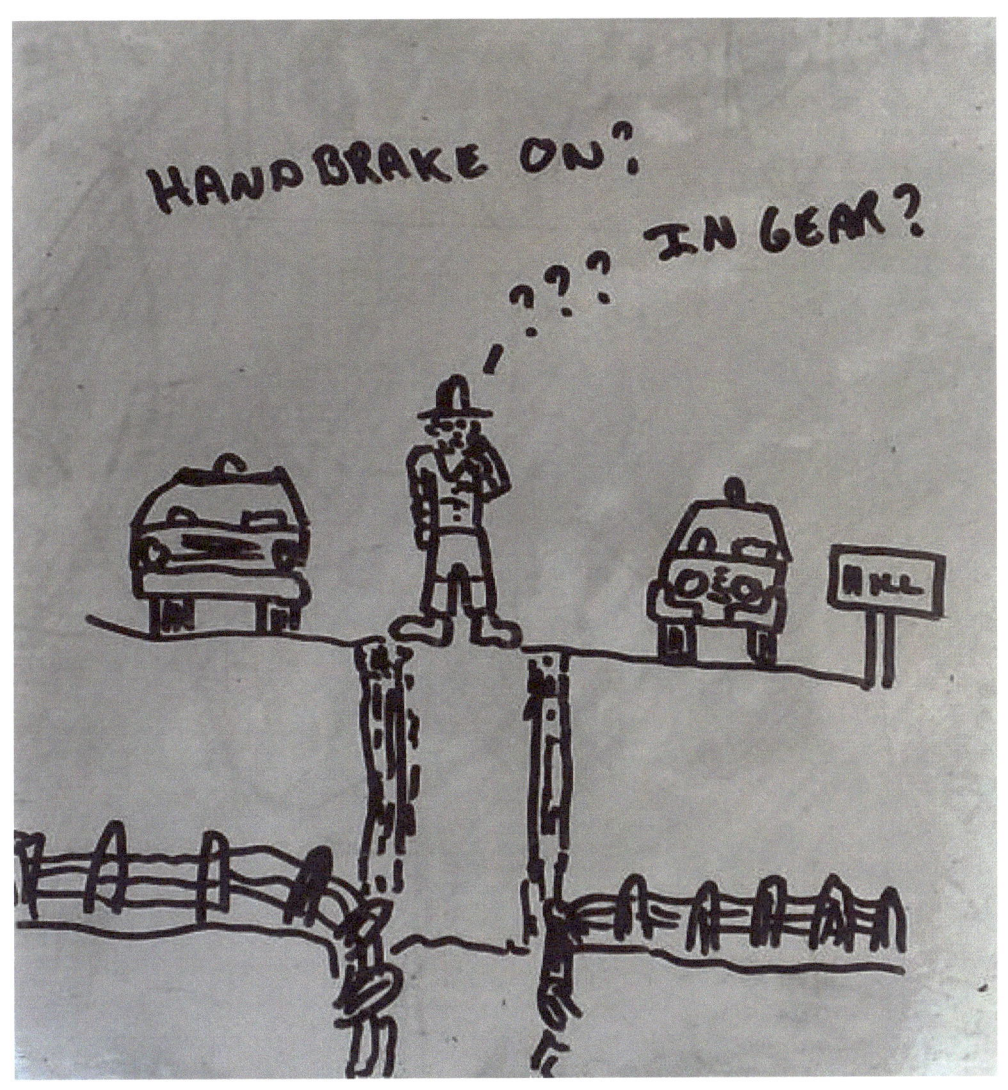

HOW MANY OF US HAVE GOTTEN OUT OF A PARKED VEHICLE AND FORGOT TO EITHER LEAVE IT IN GEAR OR THE HANDBRAKE ON?

I KNOW THAT I AM GUILTY OF THIS, ALBEIT MANY, MANY YEARS AGO, BUT I DID IT JUST THE SAME.

AND I AM SURE SO HAVE MANY OF YOU.

YOU HEAR STORIES OF CARS AND THE LIKE ROLLING DOWN HILLS AND CRASHING INTO FENCES, PEOPLE OR EVEN GETTING CLEANED UP BY OTHER VEHICLES.

SO SIMPLE YET IT IS SO EASILY FORGOTTEN. WHEN YOU PARK, MAKE SURE THAT THE HANDBRAKE IS ON AND IN GEAR.

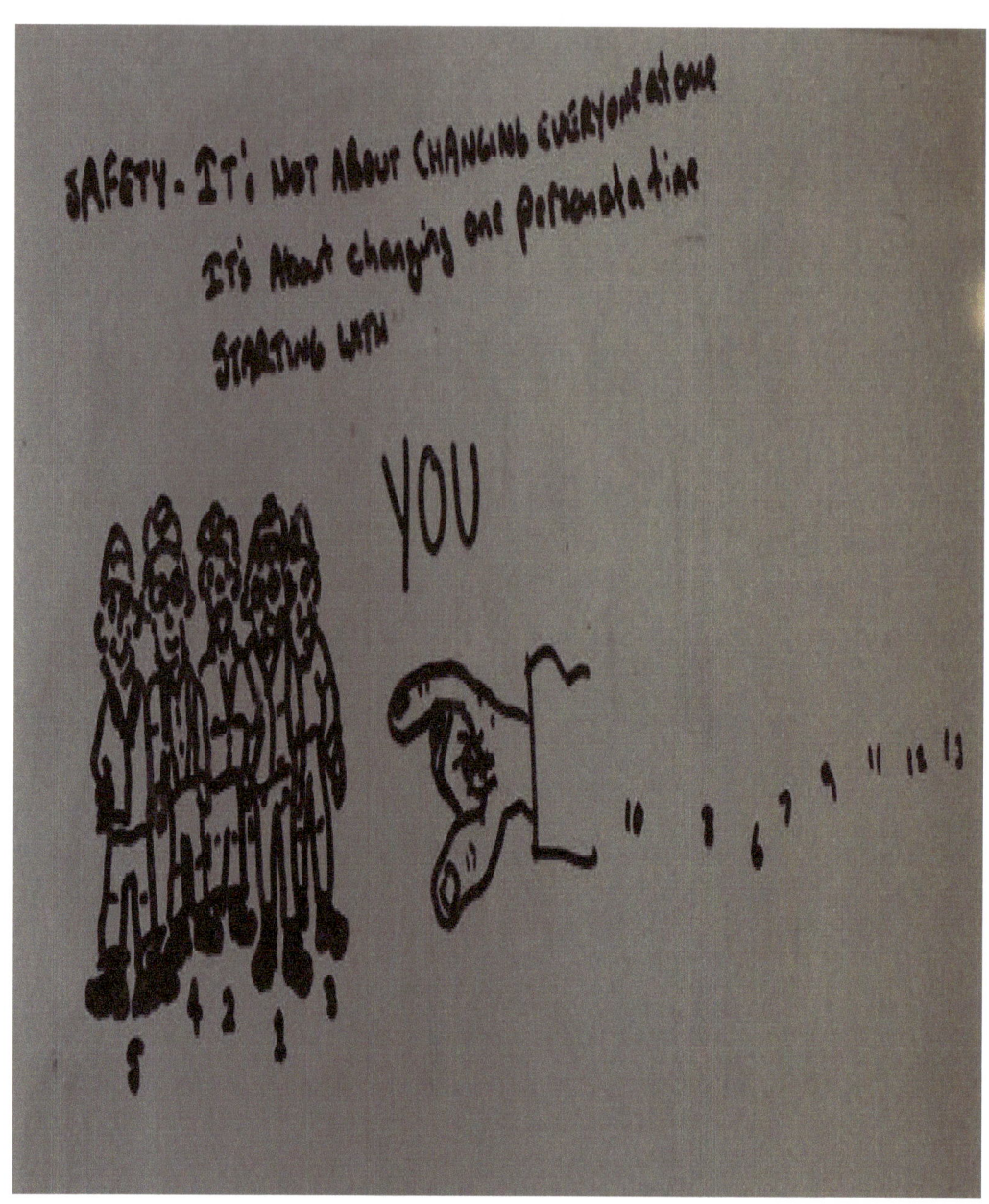

MANY PEOPLE THINK THAT BY DOING A SAFETY COURSE OR REGIME THAT YOU CAN CHANGE EVERYBODY AT ONCE, BUT THE TRUTH OF THE MATTER IS THAT THE AIM IS TO CHANGE ONE PERSONS' OUTLOOK AT A TIME AND THEN EVENTUALLY THE OTHERS WILL FOLLOW.

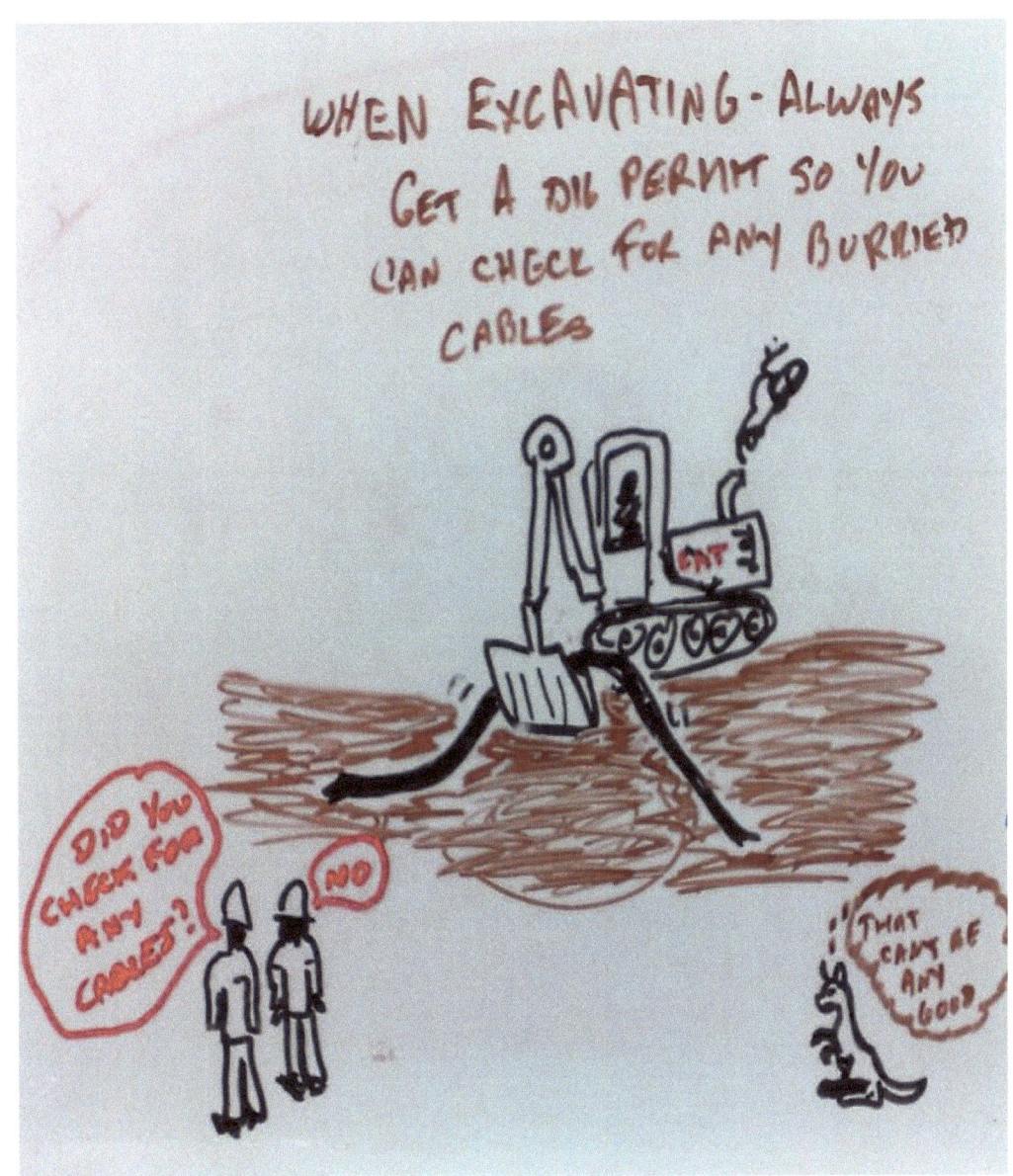

IF YOU WORK IN THE MINING GAME, AT HOME, ON ANY OTHER JOB, IF YOU ARE GOING TO EXCAVATE, THEN YOU SHOULD GET A 'DIG PERMIT' OR AT LEAST DO DUE DILIGENCE TO FIND OUT IF THERE ARE ANY BURIED CABLES OR PIPES.

OTHERWISE IT MAY TURN OUT TO BE A COSTLY EXERCISE.

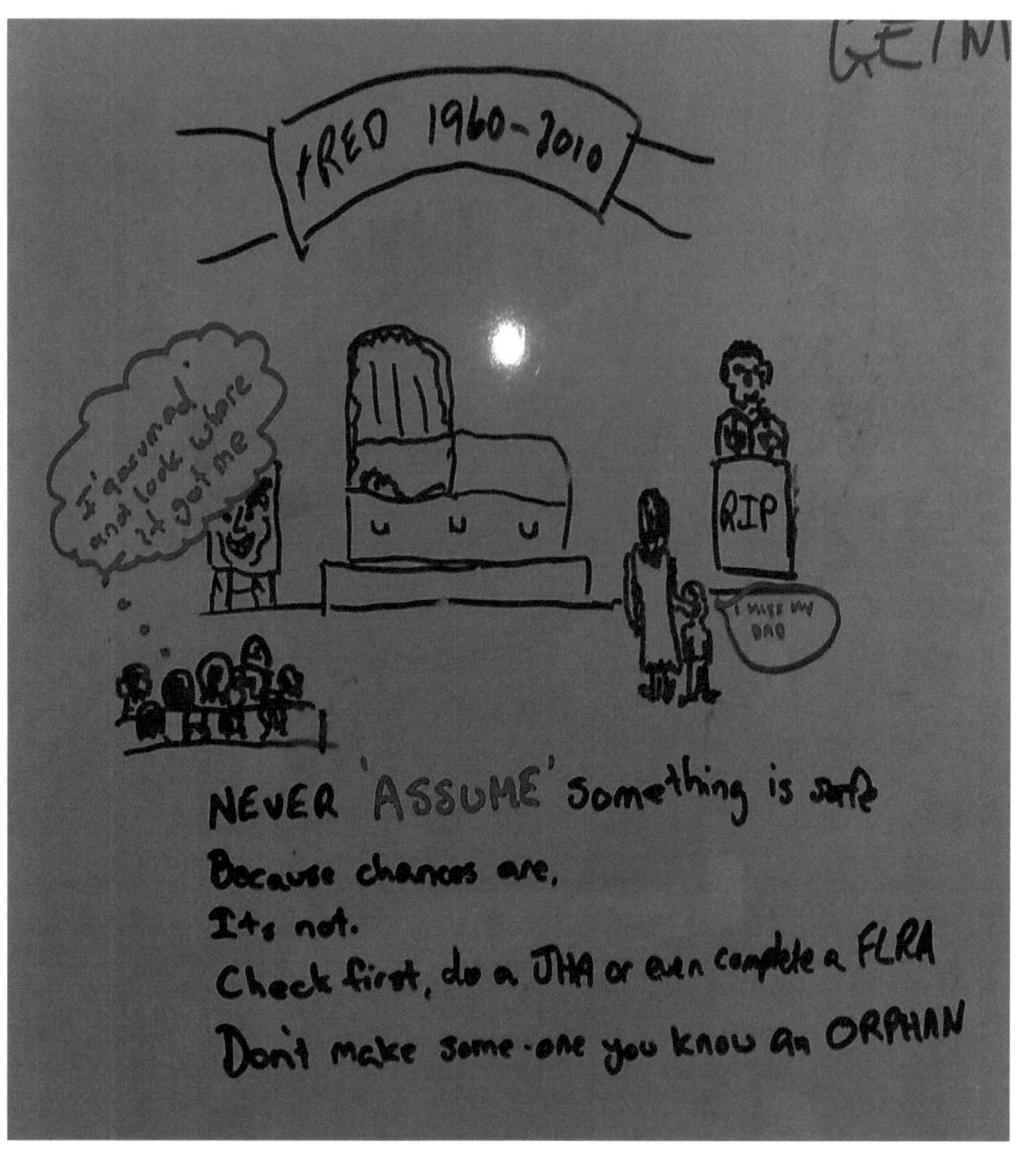

HOW OFTEN HAVE WE ALL 'ASSUMED' SOMETHING WAS CORRECT OR WRONG?

AND WE ALWAYS ARE PROVED WRONG, BECAUSE WE NEVER CHECKED THINGS OUT.

SAFETY IS NO DIFFERENT. IF WE ASSUME THAT IT IS SAFE TO DO A JOB, THEN WE HAVE NOT CHECKED AT ALL, BUT HAVE MERELY PROCEEDED TO DO 'UNSAFE' WORK, PUTTING NOT ONLY OUR LIVES IN DANGER BUT THOSE OF OTHERS AS WELL.

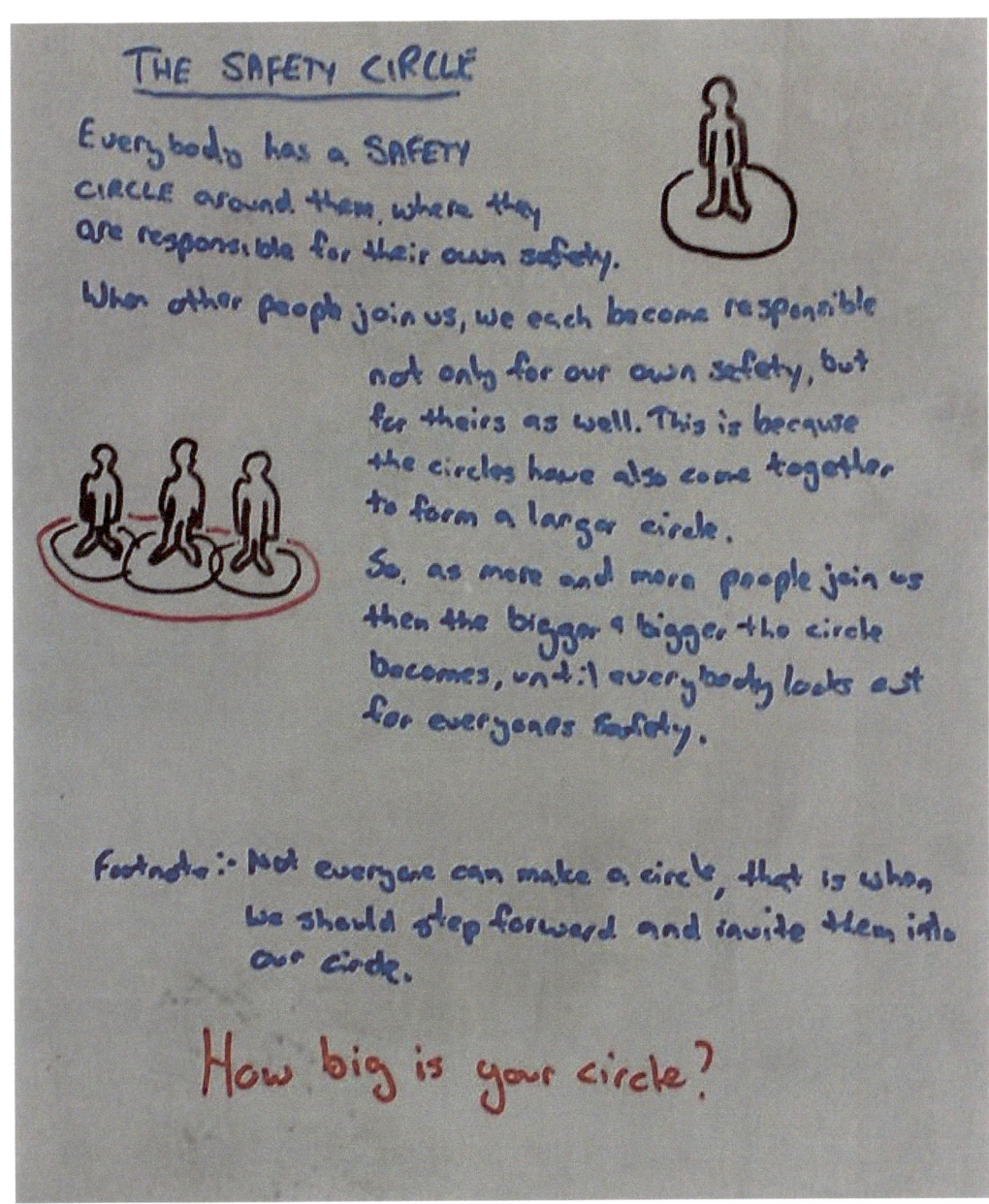

THE SAFETY CIRCLE

'THE SAFETY CIRCLE' IS AN IMPORTANT CONCEPT THAT WE MUST ALL UNDERSTAND, HENCE THE EXTRA PAGES DEDICATED TO THIS IDEA, SO THAT PEOPLE CAN GRASP THIS CONCEPT.

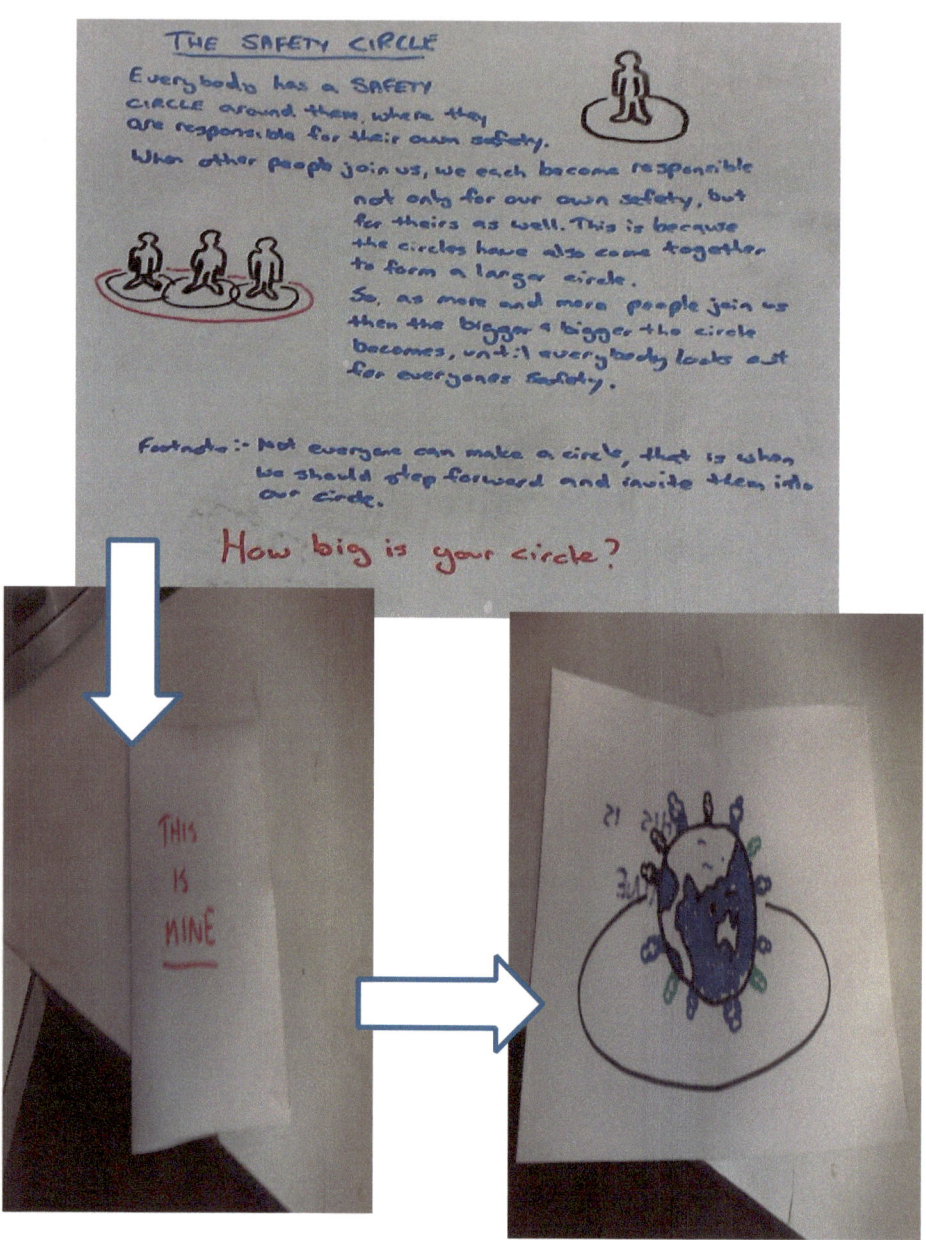

All of us have an area around us, which we consider our 'safety' zone or 'our' space. When we look after ourselves, we are really

Concentrating on looking after what is in this zone, because that way we will be safe and happy.

Safety circles, square zones, and quadratic areas of importance…what is

This guy talking about?

Well, only safety circles, anyway.

Each of us has a comfort zone which surrounds us. If people come too close to us, we feel threatened and usually step back. The same can be said for safety.

If we are unsafe, for whatever reason, then we will feel threatened and uncomfortable.

Hence, the safety circle.

When we have other people join us in the workplace, then their circle joins with ours and we both end up looking out for each other's safety and wellbeing.

And so on and so on.

The more people that join and come together means that the circles will increase in size and complexity, until everyone is covered.

Once in a while, we find that some people are unable to make a safety circle or comfort zone of their own.

When this happens, for whatever reason, then it is up to us and others to increase the size of our circle to incorporate these people.

This can include teaching them, helping them, guiding their actions, making sure that they just go home safe and in one piece.

No matter what is ever needed, we should never turn a person away from us because we were like that person, at one stage and that is how we received our help and our safety circle.

Corny? Well maybe, but if it saves lives and means looking out for each other, I know what I would prefer.

The world is my safety circle & will remain so.

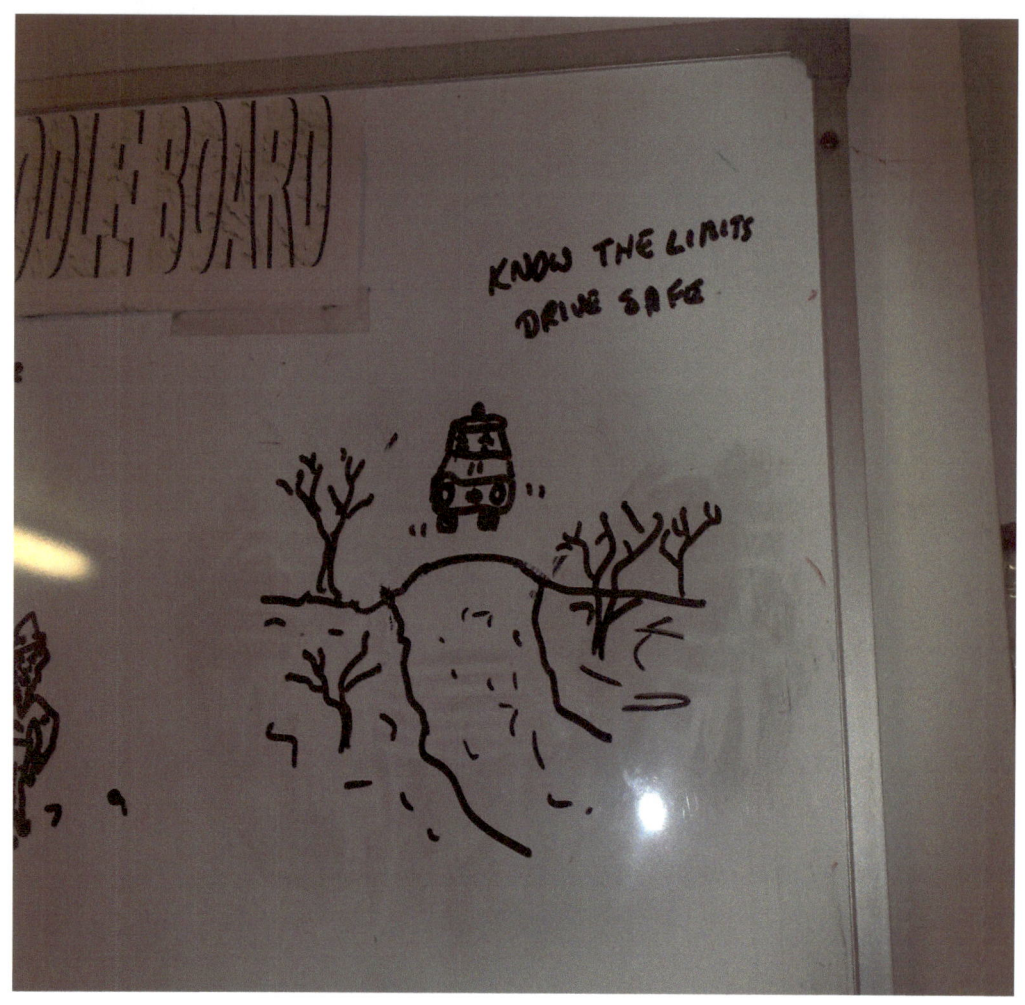

WHENEVER YOU DRIVE YOU NEED TO KNOW THE RULES CONCERNING SPEED LIMITS, CARE IN DRIVING AND MANY OTHER THINGS.

DRIVE SAFE AND YOU ARRIVE AT YOUR DESTINATION, DRIVE ANY OTHER WAY AND YOU RUN THE RISK OF NOT ONLY NOT ARRIVING, BUT CAUSING EITHER DAMAGE TO YOURSELF, OTHERS AND PROPERTY.

TEN MINUTES OF SAFER DRIVE TIME CAN EQUATE TO HOURS OF FUN FOR ALL

THE RULE OF 3

No matter what work we undertake or proceedure we implament, it has to pass the 'rule of 3'

1) Is it safe?
2) Is it practicable?
3) Is it sensible?

If it fails any of these then we must use the 3 R's

1) Re-Think what needs to be achieved
2) Re-Evaluate the hazards and work involved
3) Re-View the process as a whole

Once this has been completed then you can go back to the 'Rule of 3' and see if each of the criteria has been met.

REMEMBER

THINK SAFE - BE SAFE - STAY SAFE

"THE RULE OF 3"

THIS IS SO SIMPLE. WHEN WE HAVE A NEW PROCEDURE OR WORK RULE WE WISH TO INTRODUCE, ALL WE HAVE TO DO IS APPLY THE ABOVE MENTIONED RULE.

RETHINK – RE EVALUATE – REVIEW

SIMPLE - EASY

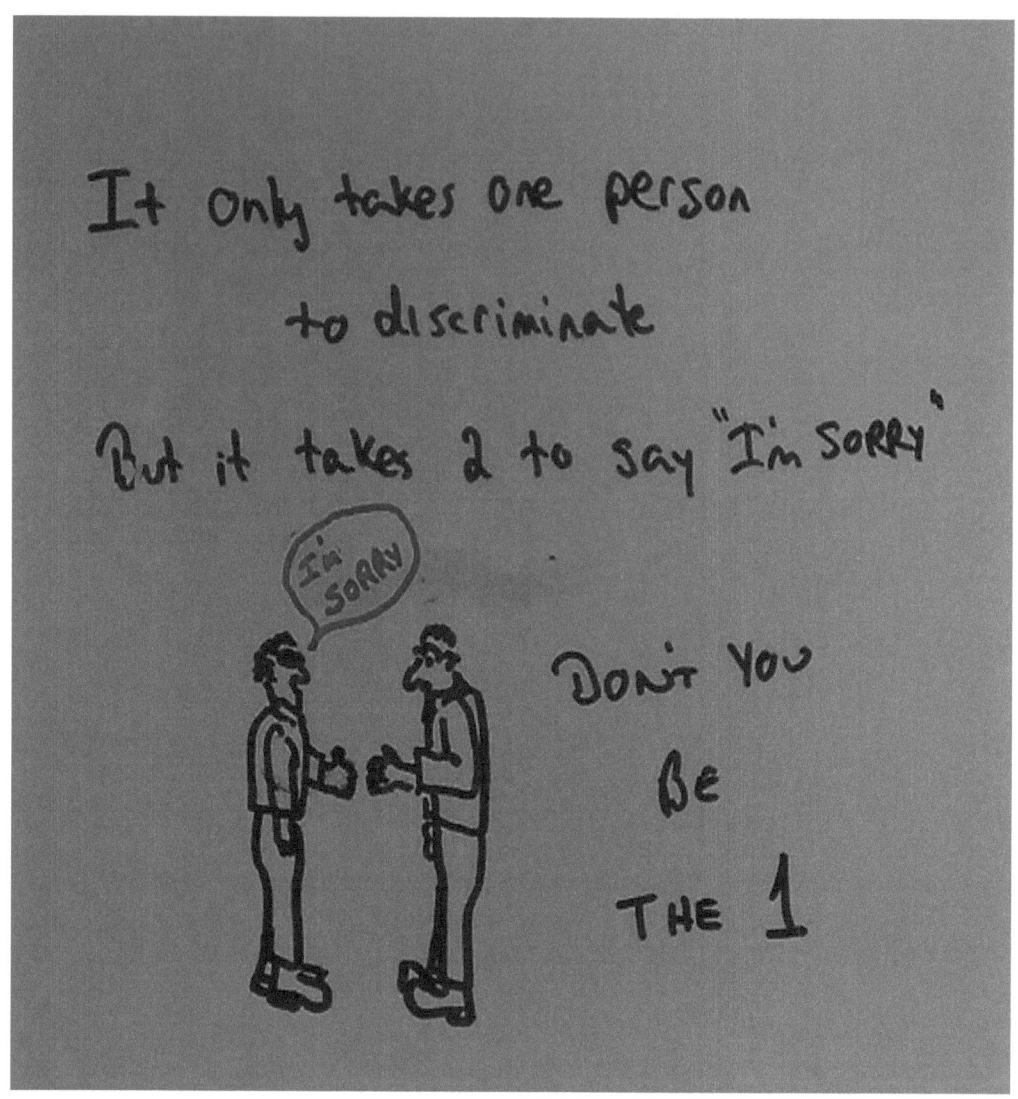

DISCRIMINATION TAKES ON A WORLD OF ITS OWN. NO MATTER WHAT RACE, RELIGION, COLOUR, LOOK, JOB, SIZE AND A MYRIAD OF OTHER CLASSIFICATIONS; DISCRIMINATION HAS NO PLACE IN TODAY'S SOCIETY.

IF WE DISCRIMINATE THEN WE DESERVE ALL THAT HAPPENS FROM THE RECRIMINATIONS FROM SUCH AN EVENT.

The world is a small place and all of us deserve to live and breathe in a world where we all show tolerance and understanding.

Imagine how we feel when we are on the receiving end.

However

In 'so saying that' we must also understand that some people are

Friends and have 'nick names' for each other. Sometimes when we hear these names called out, we are offended and immediately call attention to it by reporting it to others.

This situation is in essence wrong.

We should approach the people involved and ask them "why" they called each other like that.

It may turn out that they are very good mates or friends and they have a laugh and get some enjoyment out of the 'jibe'.

That is when we should 'step' back and accept the situation, because it is up to them, not us to say what they can 'call' each other.

If we do not accept that situation, then we run the risk of actually having 'reverse' discrimination, where we believe that everyone

Should conform to our way of thinking.

All too often we will jump on a band wagon or our high horse without thought or understanding of the why's and wherefores' of any given situation.

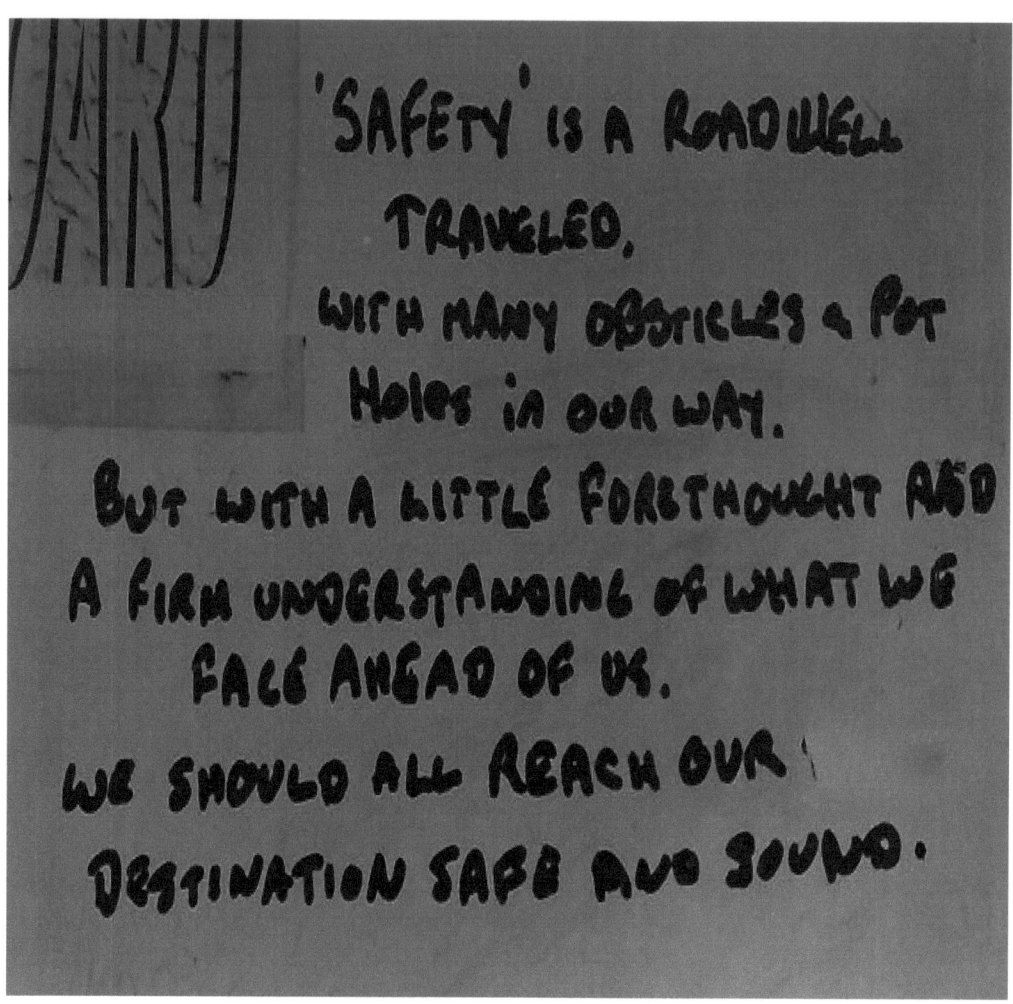

SAFETY IS A LONG ROAD AND SOME DAYS IT SEEMS TO GET LONGER AND LONGER.

ALL ANY OF US CAN DO IS TRY TO ACCEPT WHAT IS AHEAD OF US AND BEHIND, BECAUSE IF WE DON'T THEN WE RUN THE RISK OF DOING SOMETHING UNSAFE AND NOT REACHING OUR DESTINATION.

LIFE IS TOO SHORT FOR BEING UNSAFE.

JUST AS DEATH OR INJURY IS TOO LONG A ROAD TO TRAVEL.

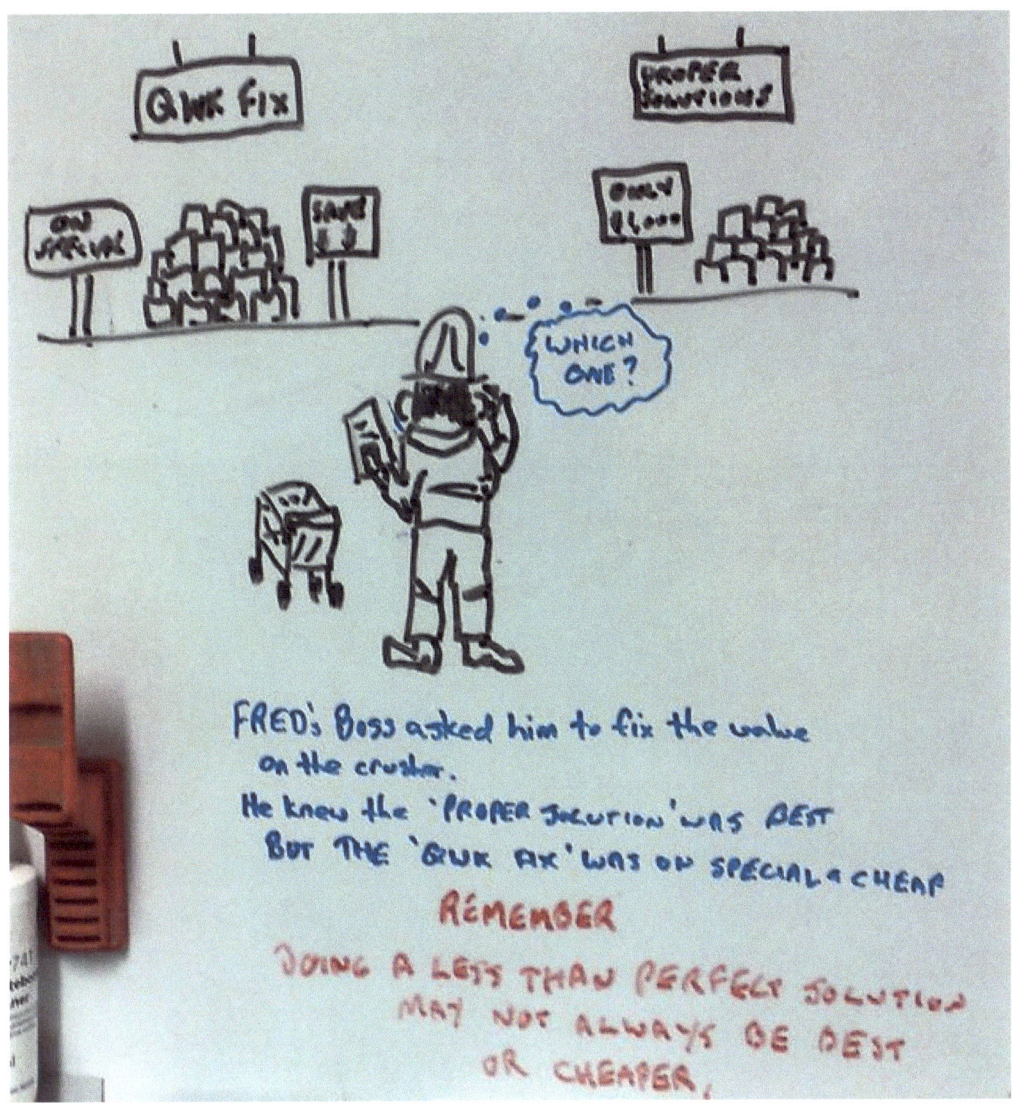

HOW OFTEN IS IT THAT EITHER AT HOME OR AT WORK WE GO FOR THE CHEAP AND QUICK SOLUTION?

IT MAY BE BECAUSE WE CAN NOT AFFORD OTHERWISE, BUT WHEN WE DO THIS, THE CHANCES ARE THAT THE MORE 'CHEAP' REPAIRS OR WORK WE HAVE DONE, THEN THE COSTLIER IT BECOMES IN THE LONG RUN.

SO TRY NOT TO FALL INTO THIS TRAP IF AT ALL POSSIBLE.

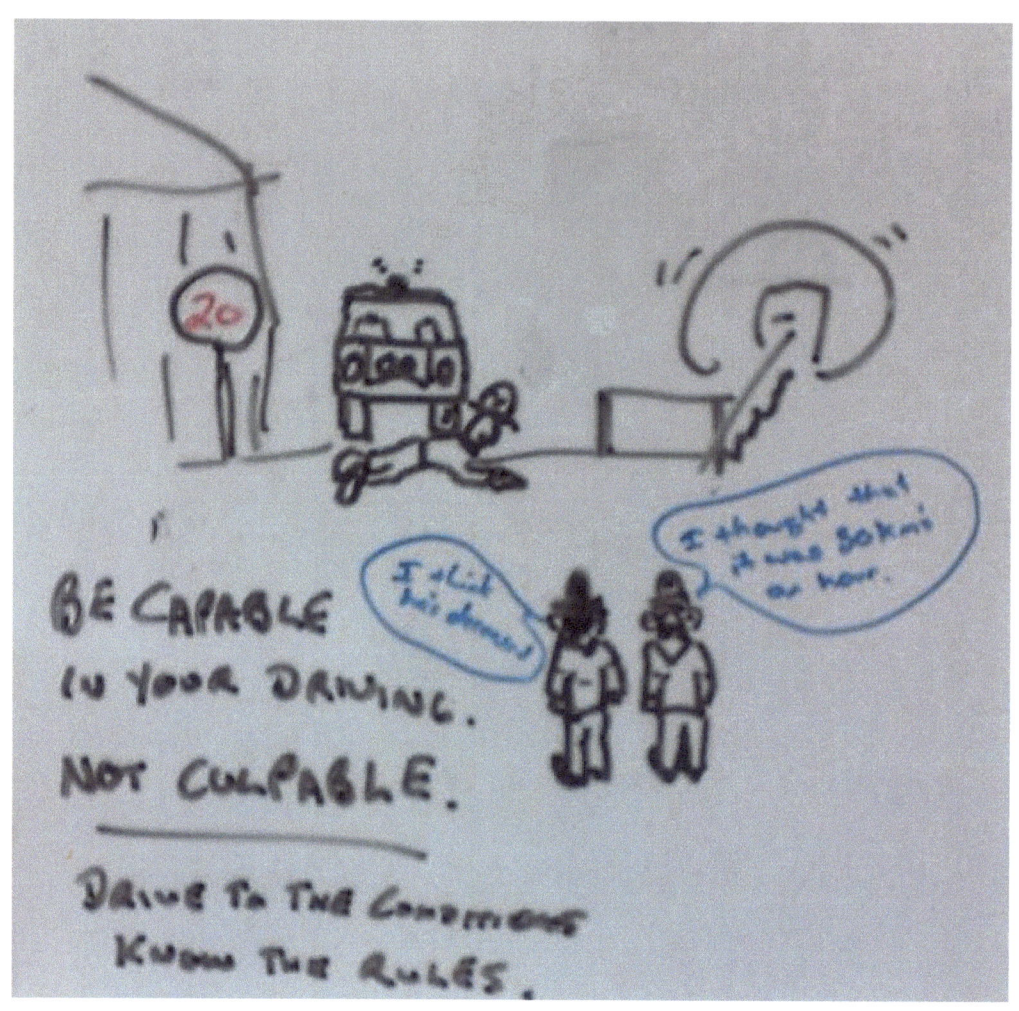

BECAUSE DRIVING MAKES UP A LARGE PROPORTION OF OUR LIVES AND ANY ACCIDENT ARISING FROM CARELESS OR IN-SENSELESS ACTS WHILE WE DRIVE, CAN HAVE FATAL AND LIFE THREATENING OUTCOMES.

NO AMOUNT OF WORDS CAN REPLACE…

DRIVE SAFE….DRIVE SENSIBLE….DRIVE TO STAY ALIVE

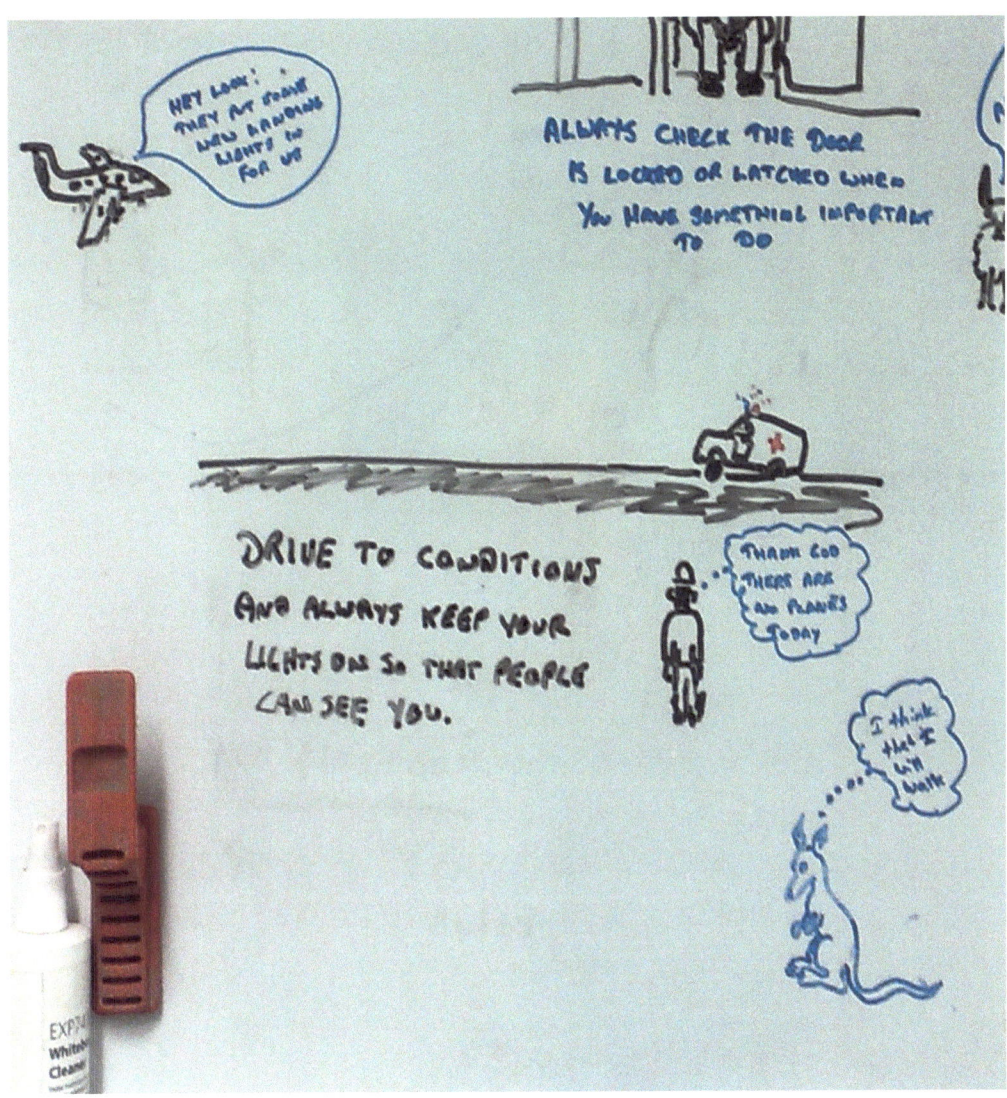

DRIVING TO THE CONDITIONS MEANS IF IT IS RAINING, SLOW DOWN; IF THE ROAD IS IN A BAD CONDITION, SLOW DOWN; IF YOU ARE UNSURE OF THE ROAD CONDITION SLOW DOWN.

EVEN IF THE ROAD CONDITION AND THE WEATHER IS FINE, THAT DOES NOT MEAN GOING AS FAST AS YOU CAN.

RESPONSIBLE DRIVING MEANS:

DRIVING SAFE

DRIVING TO KEEP THOSE AROUND YOU ALIVE AS WELL

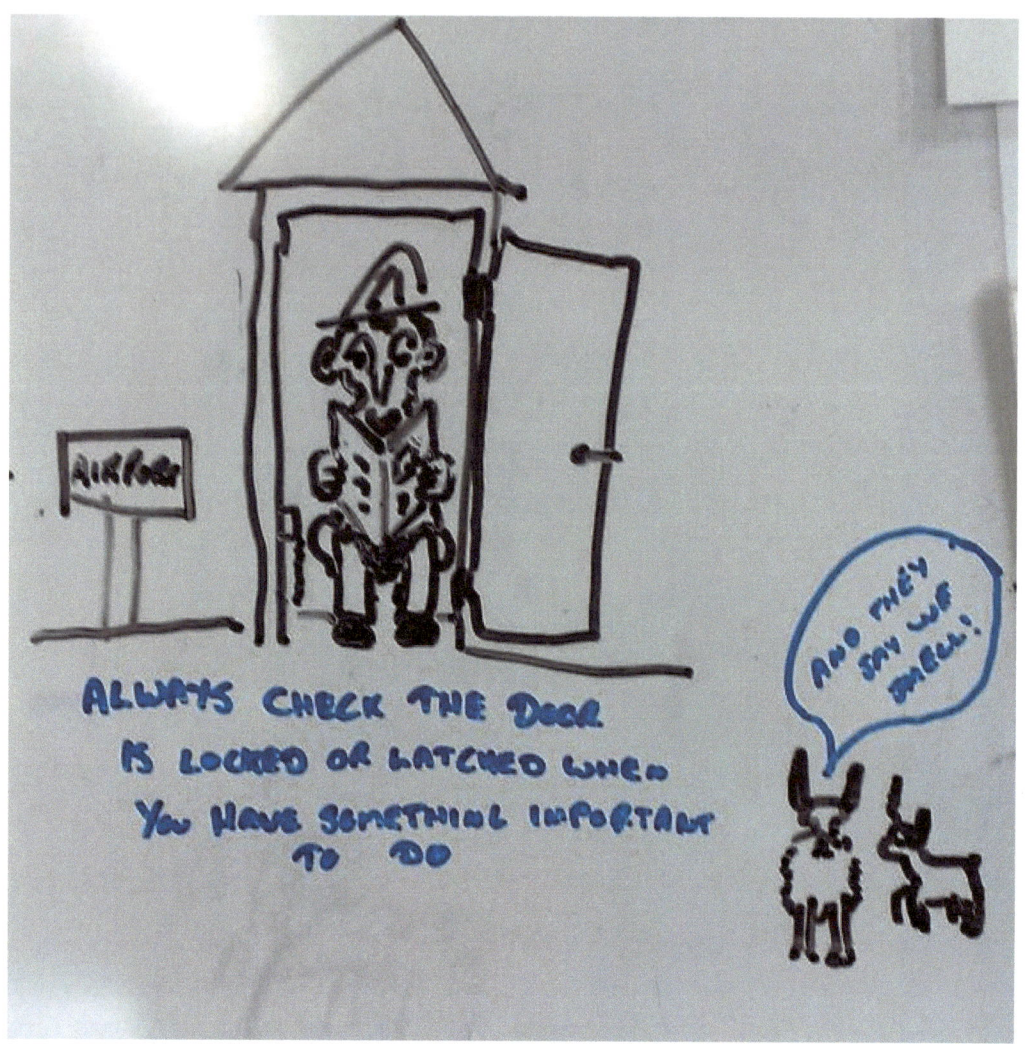

MANY TIMES, BOTH HERE IN AUSTRALIA AND AROUND THE WORLD, PEOPLE FORGET TO LOCK THEIR DOORS AND WINDOWS.

IN THE WORLD THAT WE LIVE IN TODAY, SECURITY IS PARAMOUNT.

HOW CAN WE EXPECT TO BE SAFE, WHEN WE CAN NOT EVEN REMEMBER BASIC STUFF?

IN DAYS PAST, IT WAS POSSIBLE TO LEAVE YOUR DOORS OPEN & UN-LOCKED, BUT 'SADLY' THIS HAS ALL CHANGED.

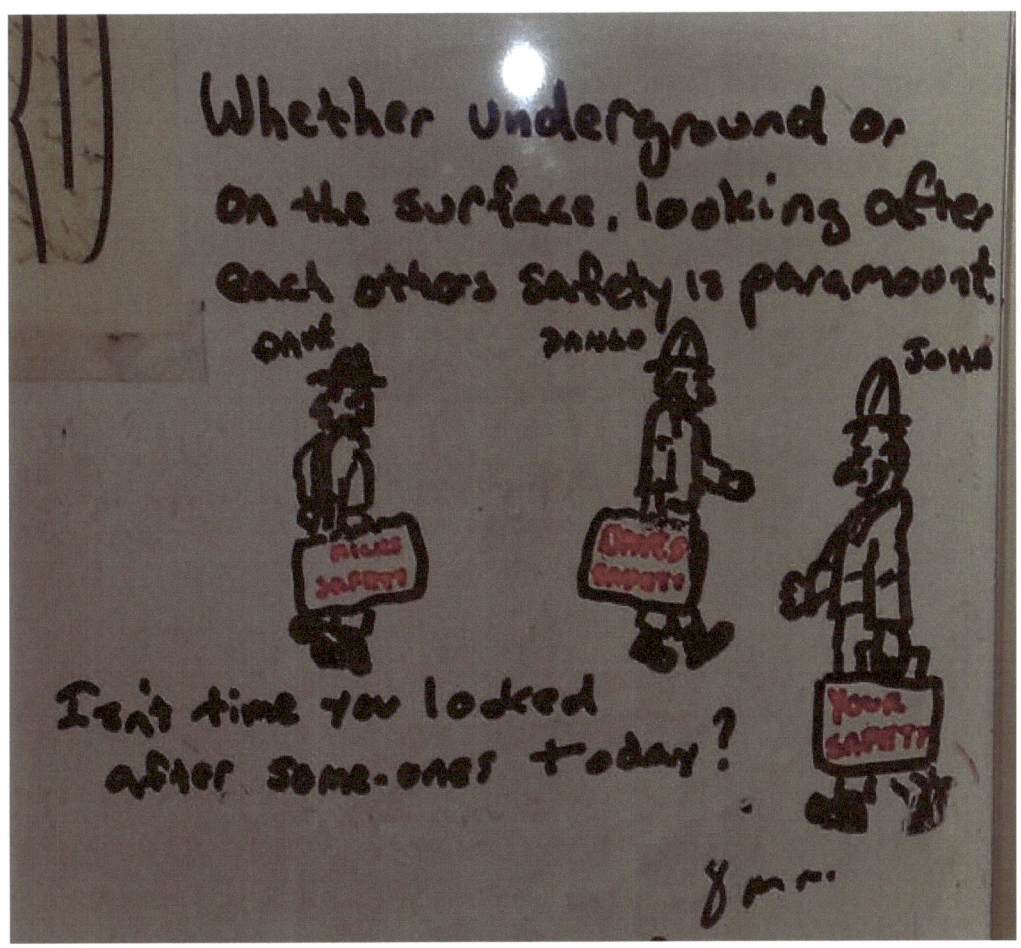

IT IS SO IMPORTANT TO LOOK AFTER EACH OTHERS SAFETY, FOR ONE SIMPLE REASON:

THEY WILL LOOK AFTER OURS.

I KNOW THIS SOUNDS 'GREEDY & MEAN', BUT IT IS TRUE, BECAUSE WE ARE HUMAN.

ALSO, AS WE WORK OR PLAY, RELYING ON OTHERS TO KEEP US SAFE MAKES ONE FEEL SAFE AND SECURE IN THE KNOWLEDGE THAT IF SOMETHING DOES GO WRONG, WE WILL HAVE HELP AND SAFETY AROUND US.

I KNOW WHAT IT IS LIKE TO SAVE SOME-ONE, SO HAVING THAT PERSON THERE CAN MAKE ALL THE DIFFERENCE.

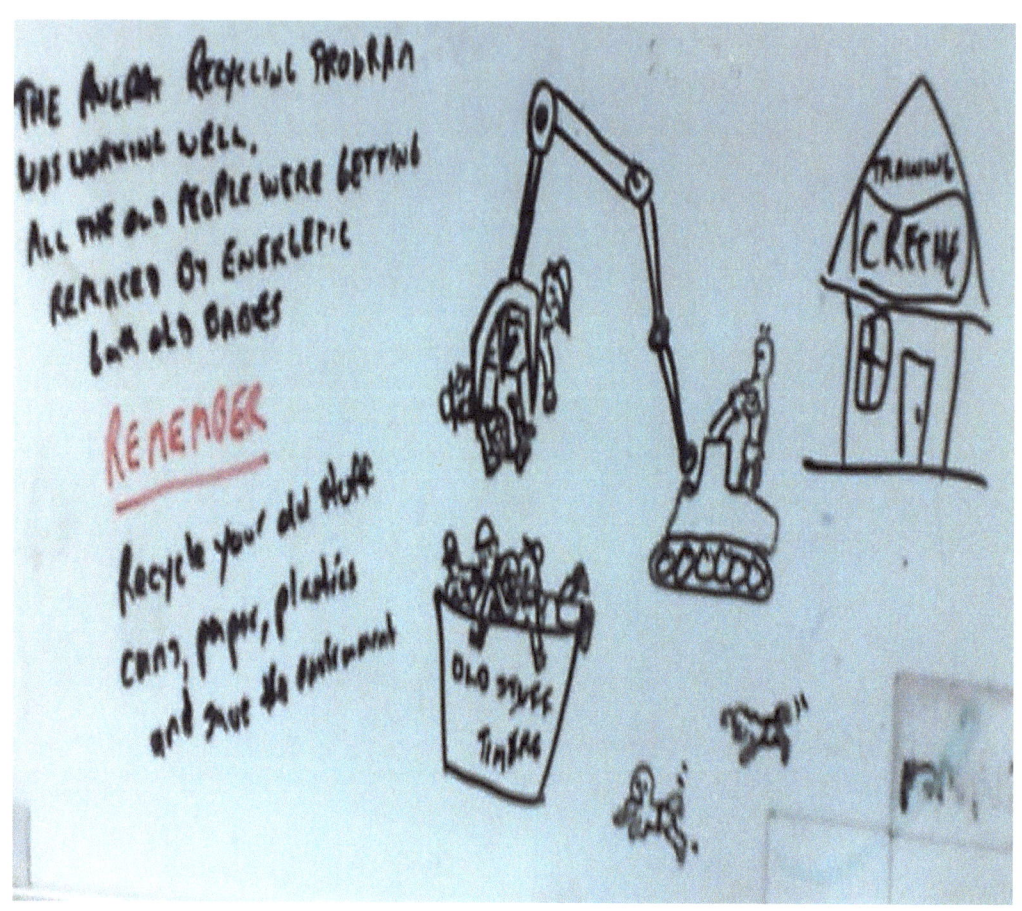

RECYCLING

IT SOUNDS SO SIMPLE, YET IT IS ANYTHING BUT.

"WHAT DO WE RECYCLE?"   "WHY" "SHOULD WE DO IT?"

WITH THE AMOUNT OF SO CALLED 'RUBBISH' THAT IS THROWN AWAY THESE DAYS, IT PAYS TO RECYCLE. RESOURCES ARE FINITE AND WE, AS THE LEADING EXPONENTS OF WASTAGE, HAVE TO TAKE RESPONSIBILITY FOR CONTRIBUTING TO THE POLLUTION OF THE PLANET.

IF WE DO NOT CLEAN UP OUR ACT, THE FINAL CURTAIN MAY COME DONE BEFORE THE PLAY IS OVER. IF IT'S OLD, RECYCLE IT… IF IT'S TO BE REPLACED, RECYCLE IT… IF IT'S TO SAVE THE ENVIRONMENT, RECYCLE IT.

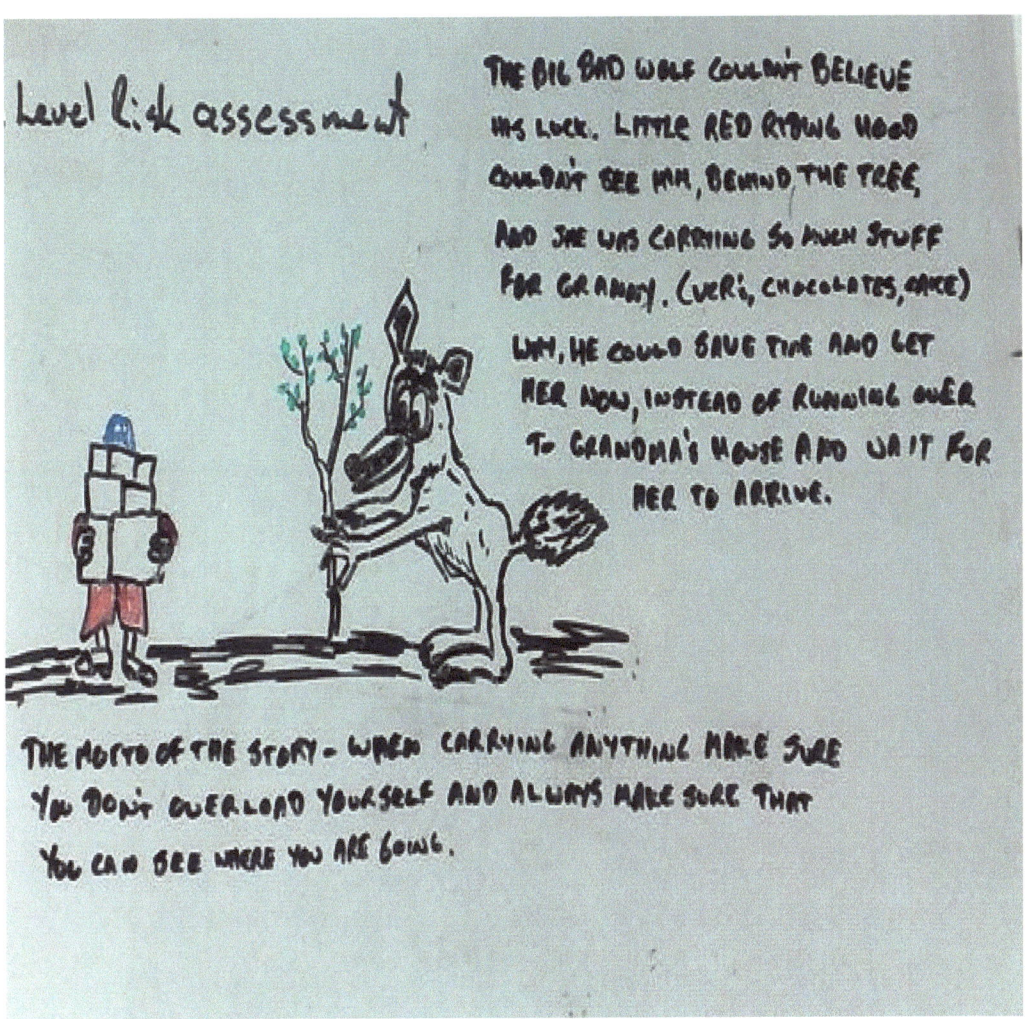

WHO HERE HAS OVERLOADED WHAT THEY CARRY?

I KNOW I HAVE, ESPECIALLY COMING BACK FROM THE SHOPS.

SO, SO EASY TO TRIP, STUMBLE, DROP GOODS, BUMP INTO PEOPLE, WHY,

BECAUSE WE HAVE NOT TAKEN CARE.

WE NEED TO KNOW WHERE WE STEP AND WHAT OUR LIMITS ARE WHEN WE CARRY ANYTHING.

IT'S NO GOOD DAMAGING OURSELVES, OTHERS, OR THE GOODS THAT WE CARRY, JUST FOR THE SAKE OF A MORE EXPEDIENT DEPARTURE AND A QUICKER DELIVERY TIME.

DON'T OVERLOAD - SEE THE WAY AHEAD

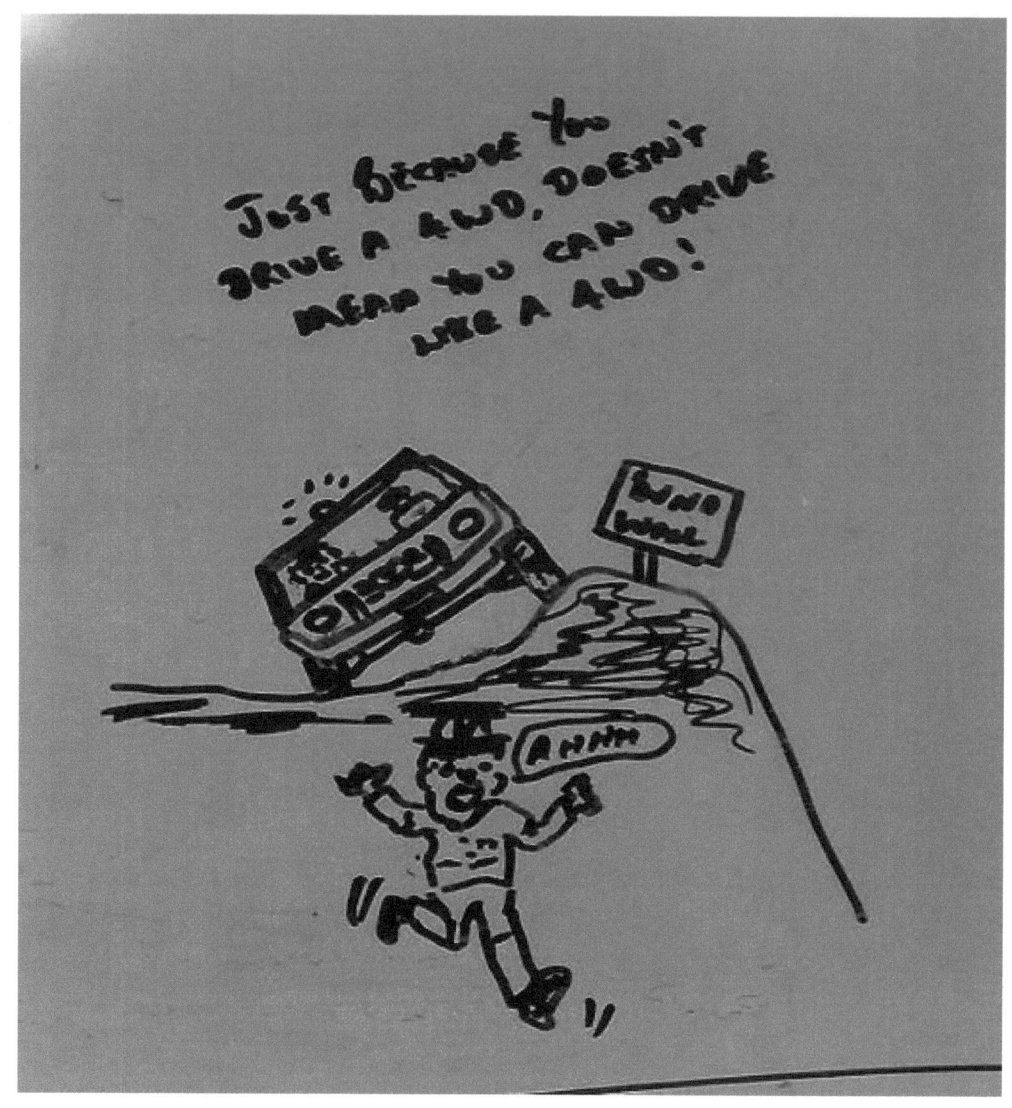

HOW OFTEN DO WE DRIVE LIKE THE CARS WE RIDE IN?

JUST BECAUSE WE DRIVE A FOUR-WHEEL- DRIVE, DOESN'T MEAN THAT WE CAN DRIVE LIKE THEY ARE MEANT FOR, OFF ROAD.

A TRUCK, LARGER CARS ETC ARE NO DIFFERENT…JUST BECAUSE THEY ARE BIGGER DOESN'T MEAN THAT WE CAN DRIVE AGGRESSIVELY OR IN A THREATENING MANNER.

DRIVE TO THE CONDITIONS - DRIVE TO THE RULES

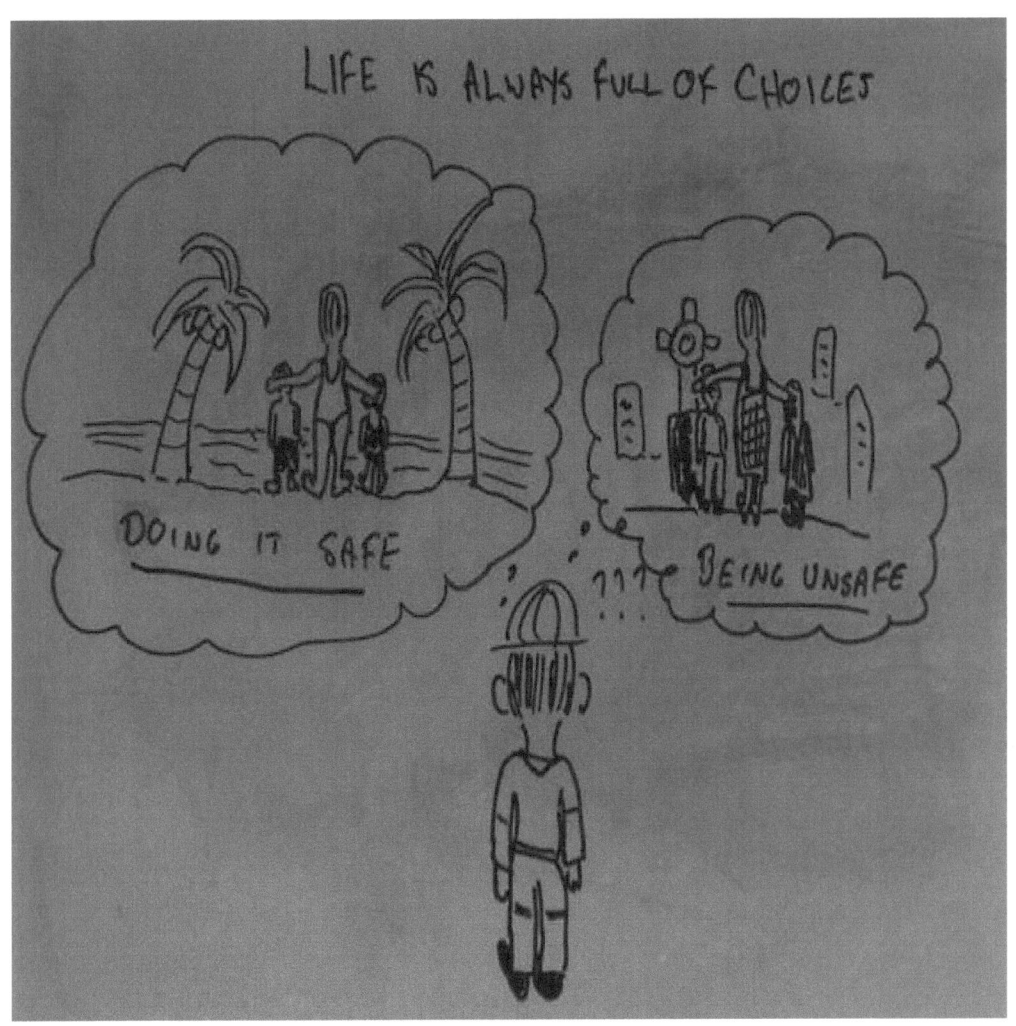

HMM…LET'S SEE. DO I CHOOSE SPENDING TIME WITH MY FAMILY OR 'SPENDING TIME WITH MY FAMILY?'

SOMETIMES WHAT WE THINK OF AS CHOICES ARE NOT REALLY CHOICES AT ALL, BUT MERELY SLACKNESS ON OUR PARTS TO AN ADVERSE 'WORK' ETHIC.

MAYBE WE WANT TO FINISH WORK EARLY AND TAKE THE EASY ROUTE, OR WE MAY BE UNDER THE PUMP TO FINISH AT AN EARLIER TIME SO THAT PRODUCTION CAN GET STARTED AGAIN.

WHATEVER…THERE IS NO CHOICE IN MY BOOK.

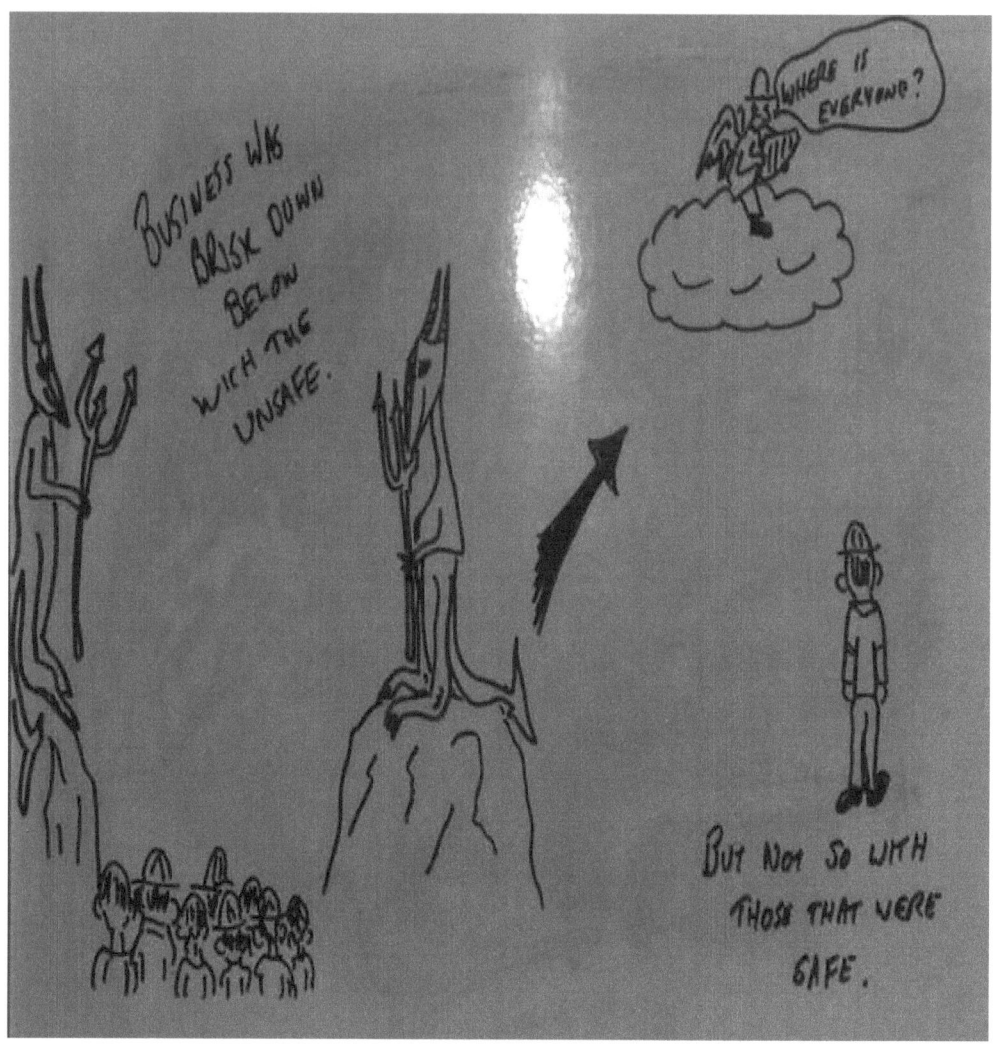

JUST AS THERE ARE DEATHS FROM BEING SAFE SO THERE ARE DEATHS FROM BEING UN-SAFE.

UNFORTUNATELY I BELIEVE THAT THE UNSAFE OUT WEIGHS THE SAFE.

WHY?...BECAUSE IF YOU ARE UNSAFE, YOU WILL CUT CORNERS, YOU WILL TAKE GREATER RISKS, YOU WILL JEOPARDIZE OTHER PEOPLES LIVES.

IN THE END IT'S UP TO YOU TO DECIDE IF YOU CAN LIVE WITH THE POSSIBILITY THAT YOU MAY HURT SOME-ONE YOU WORK WITH OR MAYBE SOME-ONE YOU CARE ABOUT.

UNSAFE - NO WAY

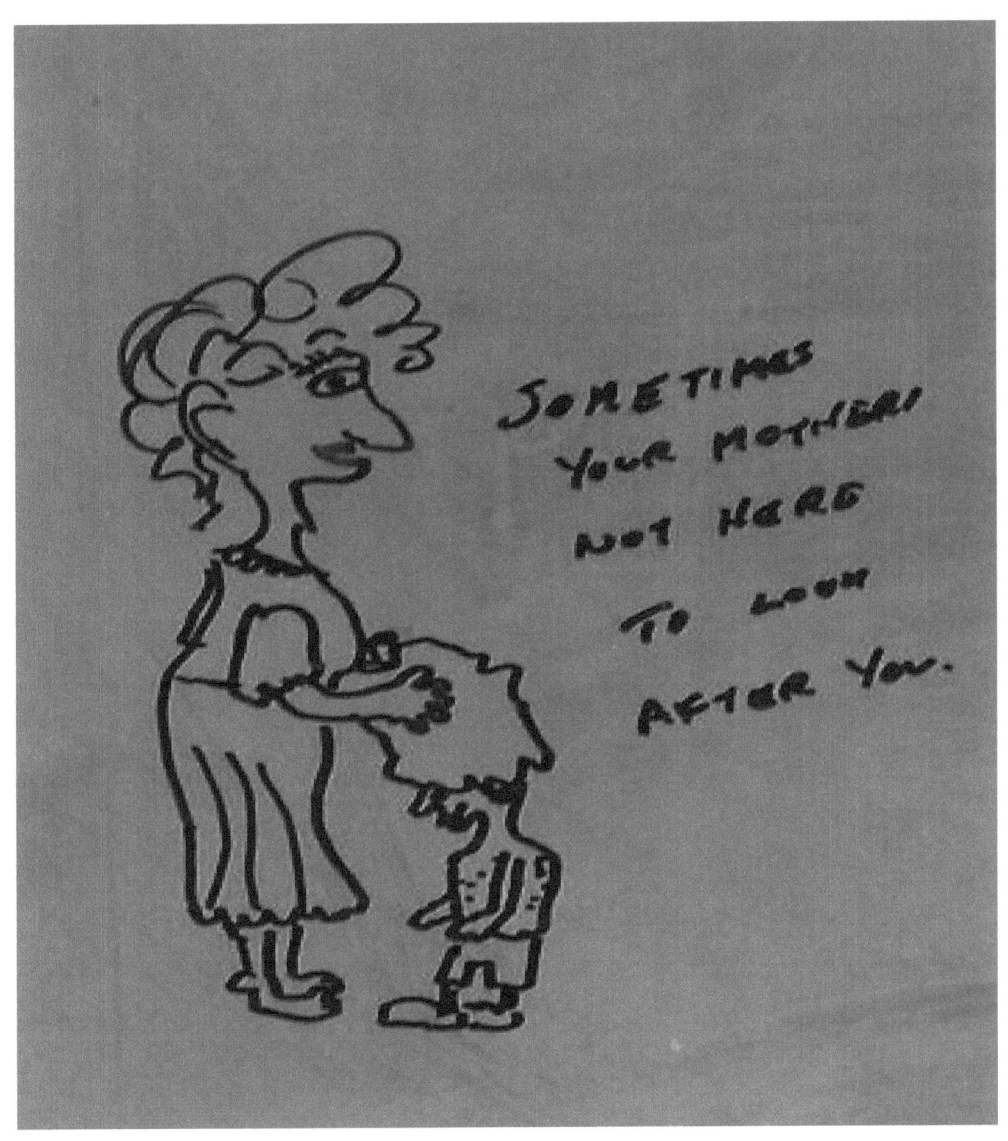

IT'S ALL TRUE.

ONCE YOU TAKE PEOPLE AWAY FROM THEIR HOME ENVIRONMENT THEIR MENTALITY DOES CHANGE, ESPECIALLY IF THEY RECEIVE EVERYTHING FROM THEIR EMPLOYERS, AT NO COST TO THEMSELVES.

THEY FORGET THAT WE ALL WORK FOR THE SAME REASON, JUST AS THEY FORGET THE BASICS IN RESPECT.

IF YOU DROP IT PICK IT UP!

IF YOU USE IT…REPLACE IT!

IF YOU RESPECT YOURSELF…YOU ALREADY DO IT!!

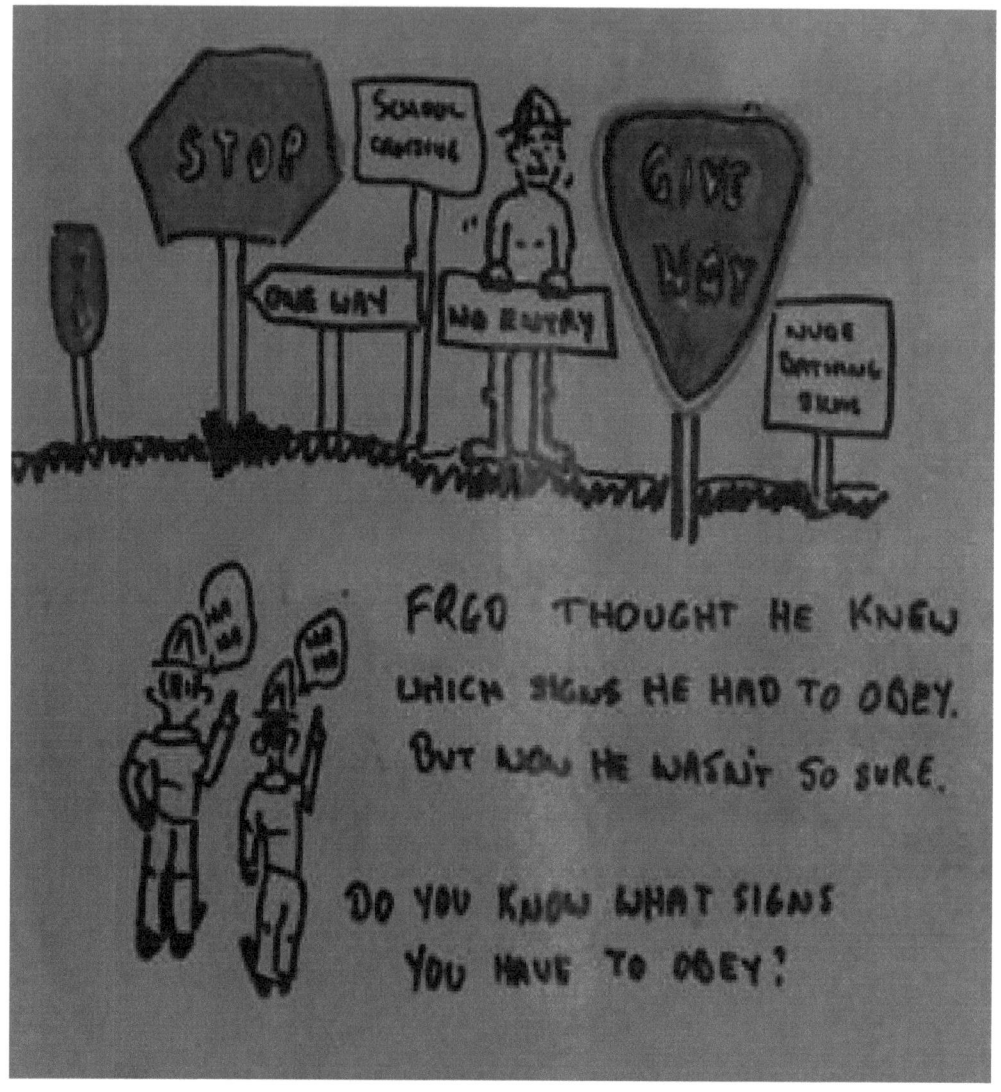

ROAD SIGNS, ADVISORY SIGNS, INFORMATION SIGNS, COMPULSORY SIGNS AND THE LIST GOES ON AND ON.

SOMETIMES IT IS QUITE HARD TO WORK OUT WHICH ONES YOU NEED TO ADHERE TO AND THOSE WHICH YOU DO NOT HAVE TO OBEY, TO THE LETTER OF THE LAW, ANYWAY.

BUT, WE MUST ALL KNOW THEM AND UNDERSTAND WHY THEY ARE IN PLACE.

IF WE DON'T WE RUN THE RISK OF HURTING OTHERS AND OURSELVES.

SO REMEMBER, IF YOU DON'T KNOW THE SIGNS, TAKE TIME OUT TO FIND OUT WHAT THEY MEAN.

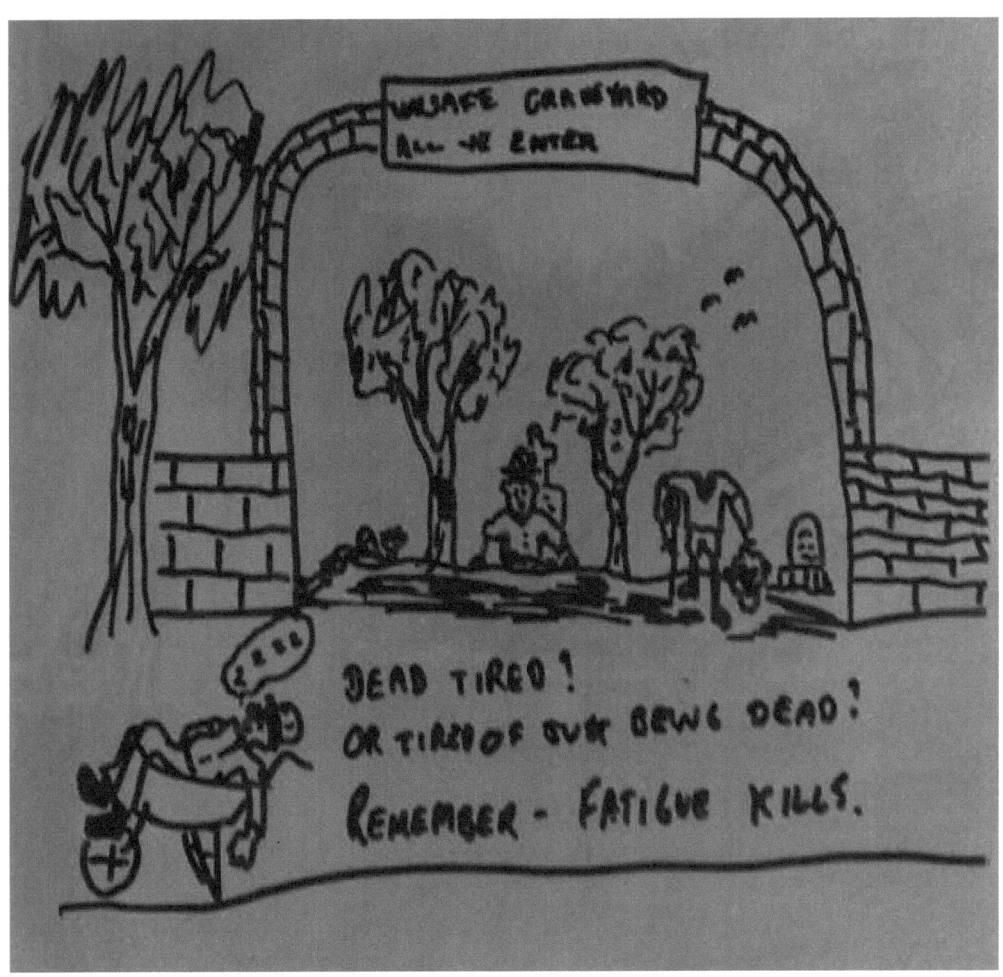

FATIGUE DOES KILL AND SO DO PEOPLE.

DRIVING TIRED, OPERATING EQUIPMENT, TRYING TO THINK WITH A SENSIBLE THOUGHT WHILE YOU ARE FATIGUED IS LIKE PARTICIPATING IN THE RUN WITH THE   BULLS. YOU MAY GET HURT, MAYBE NOT.

HOW MANY CAR ACCIDENTS HAVE WE HEARD ABOUT BECAUSE THE DRIVER FELL ASLEEP AT THE WHEEL?

HOW MANY TIMES HAVE WE OURSELVES FALLEN ASLEEP WHILE SITTING IN AN ARM CHAIR, EVEN THOUGH WE WANTED TO STAY AWAKE AND WATCH SOMETHING ON TV?

FATIGUED? TAKE A QUICK NAP. REFRESH, REPLENISH WHAT SLEEP DEPRAVATION HAS TAKEN AWAY.

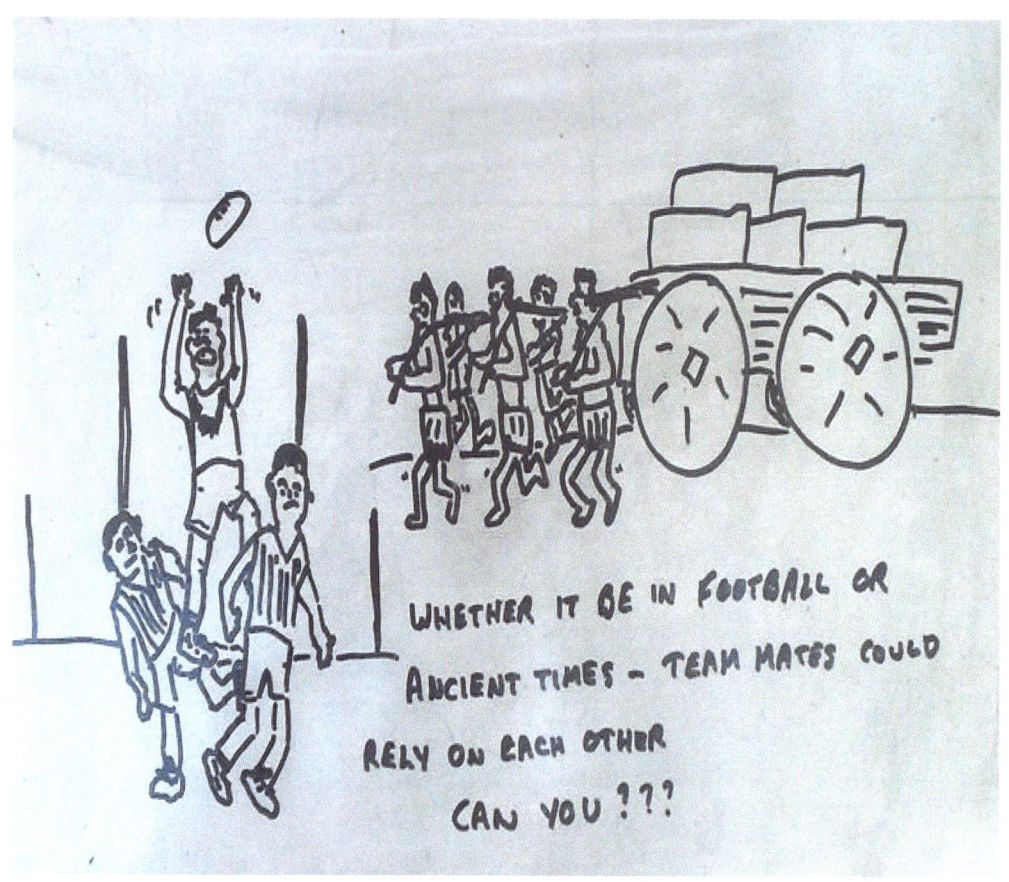

WE ALL RELY ON SOME OTHER PERSON, WHETHER WE LIKE TO ADMIT IT OR NOT. MOST OF THE TIME IT IS A LOVED ONE OR FAMILY. OTHER TIMES IT IS OUR WORK MATES OR THOSE WE SOCIALISE WITH.

MOST OF THE TIME THE SUPPORT NEEDED IN ALL THE CASES IS GENERALLY THE SAME.

WE WANT SUPPORT. WE WANT UNDERSTANDING. WE WANT TO BE PART OF A TEAM ENVIRONMENT. WE WANT TO FEEL SAFE.

AFTER ALL, IT IS OUR COMFORT ZONE.

WHY? BECAUSE WE ARE PART OF THAT RACE WHICH IS CALLED BEING HUMAN.

IF SOME-ONE NEEDS HELP, GIVE IT TO THEM. MAKE THEM FEEL SAFE AND SECURE, OTHERWISE YOU WILL MAKE THEM FEEL ALONE, VULNERABLE AND NSAFE.

NO-ONE WANTS THAT.

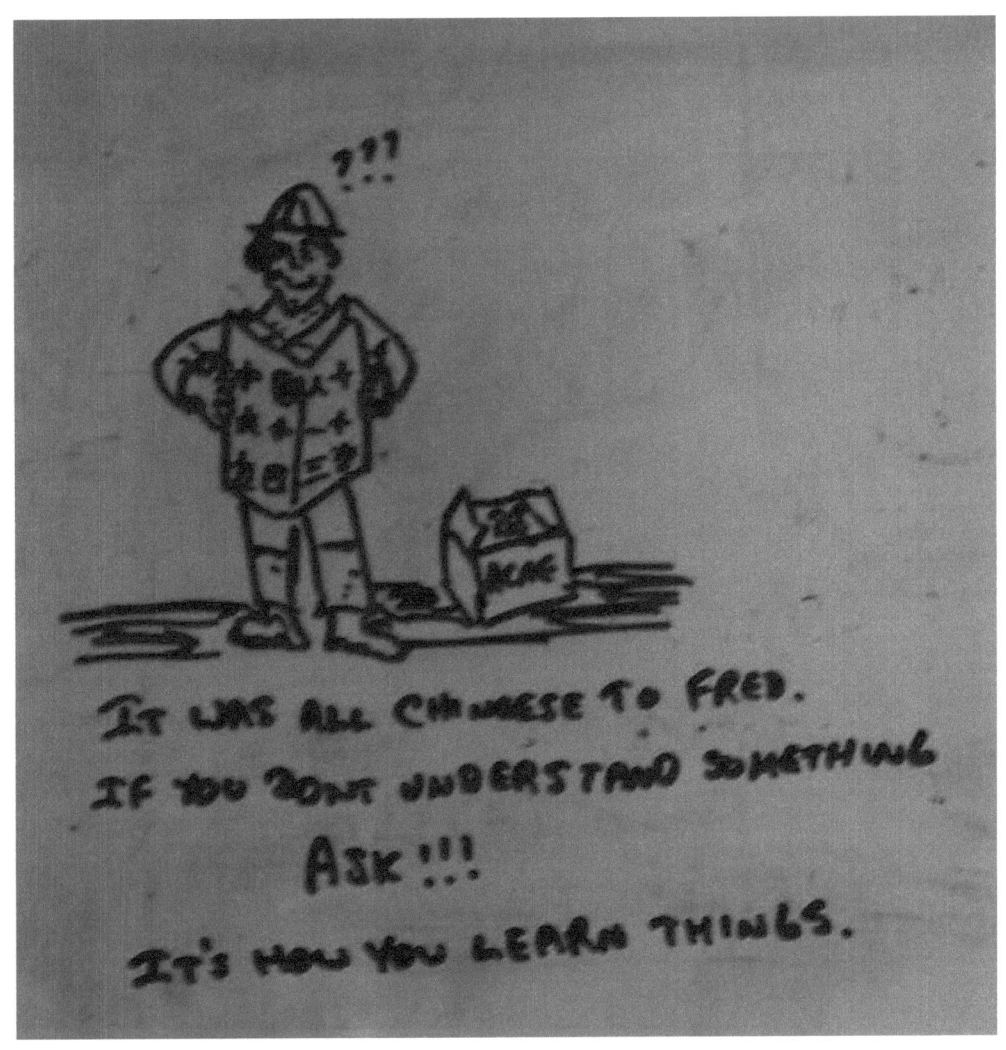

HOW MANY TIMES HAVE WE ALL TRIED TO READ OR LISTEN TO THE INSTRUCTIONS, ONLY TO FIND THAT WE HAVE NOT REALLY NDERSTOOD AT ALL?

THAT IS WHEN WE SHOULD ASK SOMEBODY, "WHAT'S IT ALL ABOUT".

BUT UNFORTUNATELY THERE IS A STIGMATISM ABOUT 'ASKING' FOR HELP IN UNDERSTANDING SOMETHING.

IF WE ASK, THEN WE MUST EITHER BE 'STUPID' OR 'NOT GOOD AT OUR JOBS', BUT THE TRUTH OF THE MATTER IS THAT ASKING FOR GUIDANCE SHOWS THAT WE WISH TO UNDERSTAND FURTHER

AND THE MORE WE UNDERSTAND, THE MORE WE LEARN AND THE MORE WE CAN HELP EACH OTHER.

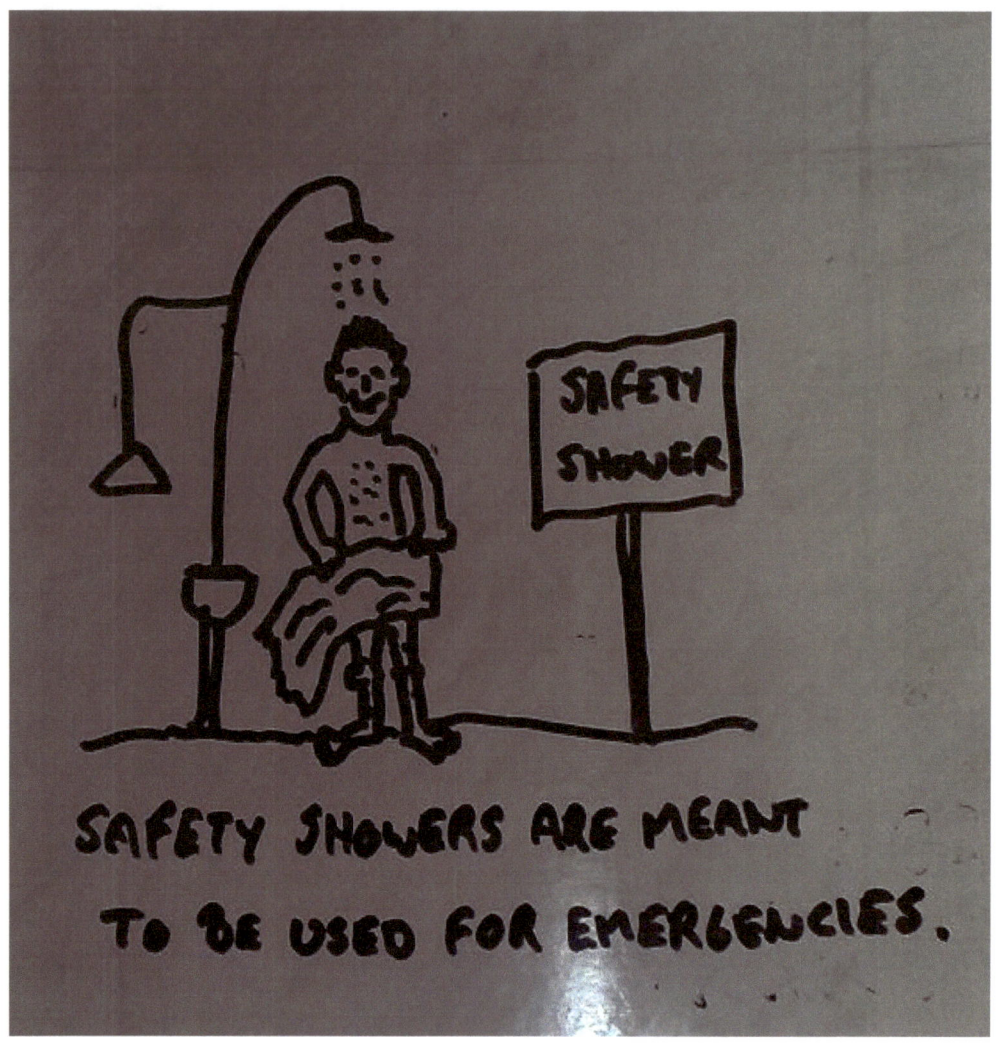

AT MANY MINES AND SOME LARGER FACTORIES YOU MAY FIND SAFETY SHOWERS.

THESE ARE USED FOR EMERGENCIES WHERE SOME-ONE MAY BE COVERED IN CONTAMINATES SUCH AS OIL, CHEMICALS, DUST ETC.

THE SHOWERS SHOULD BE USED SOLELY FOR EMERGENCY SITUATIONS AND NOT FOR EVERYDAY USES.

THEY SHOULD ALSO BE SERVICED REGULARLY AND THE WATER SHOULD BE OF ACCEPTABLE QUALITY.

RUNOFF FROM THESE SHOWERS COULD AND SHOULD BE ALSO A PRIORITY.

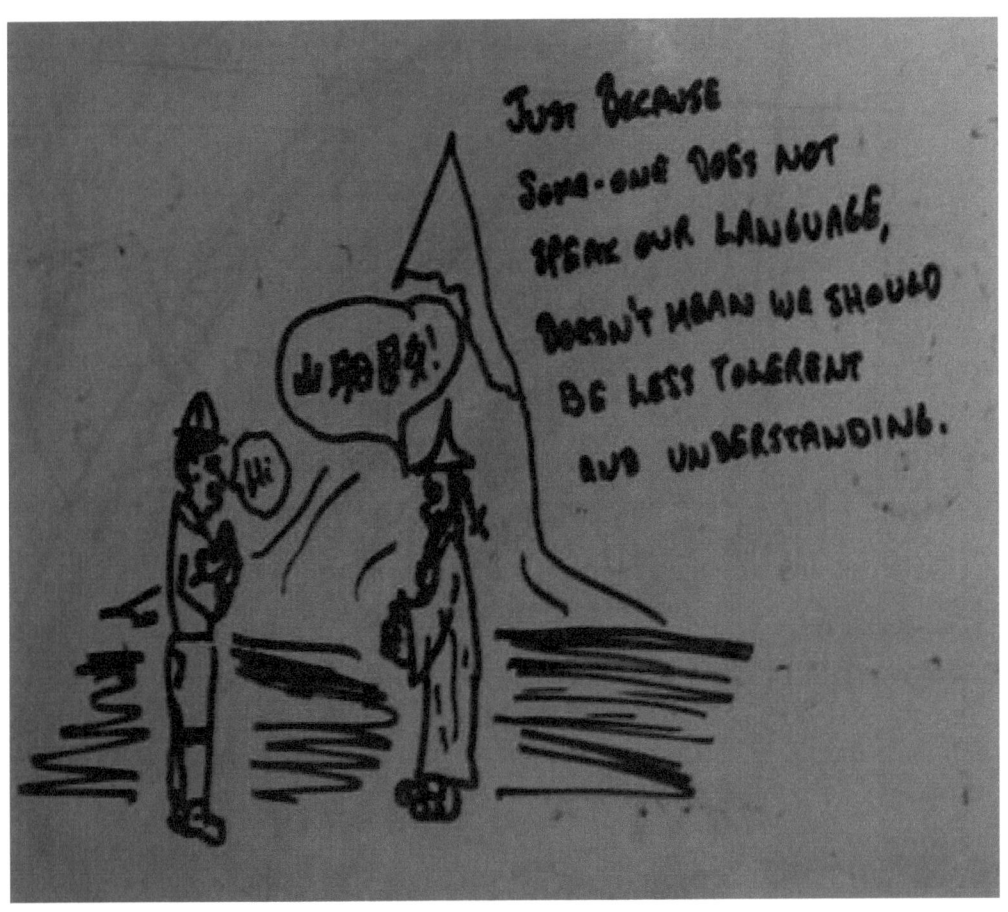

AGAIN WITH THIS DRAWING WE COME BACK TO THE AGE OLD FEELINGS THAT

PEOPLE HAVE TOWARDS OTHERS WHO DO NOT SPEAK OUR LANGUAGE OR ACT AS WE DO.

THE REVERSE IS ALSO TRUE.

WE DO NOT KNOW THEIR LANGUAGE LET ALONE UNDERSTAND THEIR CULTURE, BUT YET WE WANT THEM TO UNDERSTAND AND SPEAK OURS.

PEOPLE NEED TO BEGIN TO ACCEPT THAT THE WORLD IS GETTING SMALLER, WITH THE ADVENT OF FASTER TRAVEL AND COMMUNICATIONS.

ALL OF US SHOULD TAKE TIME OUT TO GET TO KNOW ONE ANOTHER, WHETHER IT BE IN OUR COUNTRY OR THEIRS.

BETTER TOLERANCE & LEARNING MEANS BETTER TEAM SPIRIT & UNDERSTANDING.

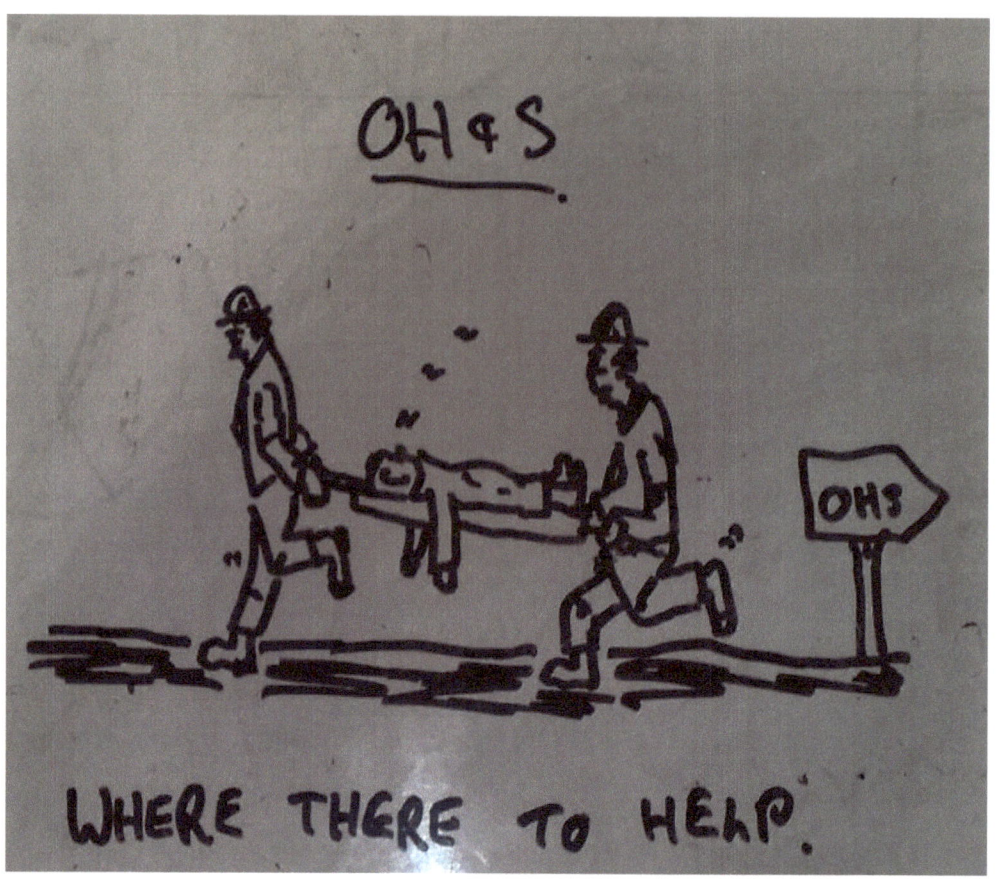

THAT'S RIGHT OH & S OR 'OCCUPATIONAL HEALTH & SAFETY' ARE THERE TO HELP YOU IN A VARIETY OF CIRCUMSTANCES.

FROM HAVING A SPLINTER, TO CUTTING A FINGER OR EVEN HAVING A BOUT OF

THE FLU, THEY ARE THERE TO HELP YOU GET BETTER.

THERE'S NOTHING WORSE THAN FEELING SICK ON SITE.

IN MOST CASES, IN MINES ANYWAY, THERE MAY BE NO DOCTORS, BUT WE STILL HAVE REGISTERED NURSES OR PARAMEDICS ON HAND TO RENDER ASSISTANCE.

IF YOU NEED HELP GO AND SEE THEM.

IF YOU NEED SOME-ONE TO TALK TO:-

THEY'RE THERE FOR YOU.

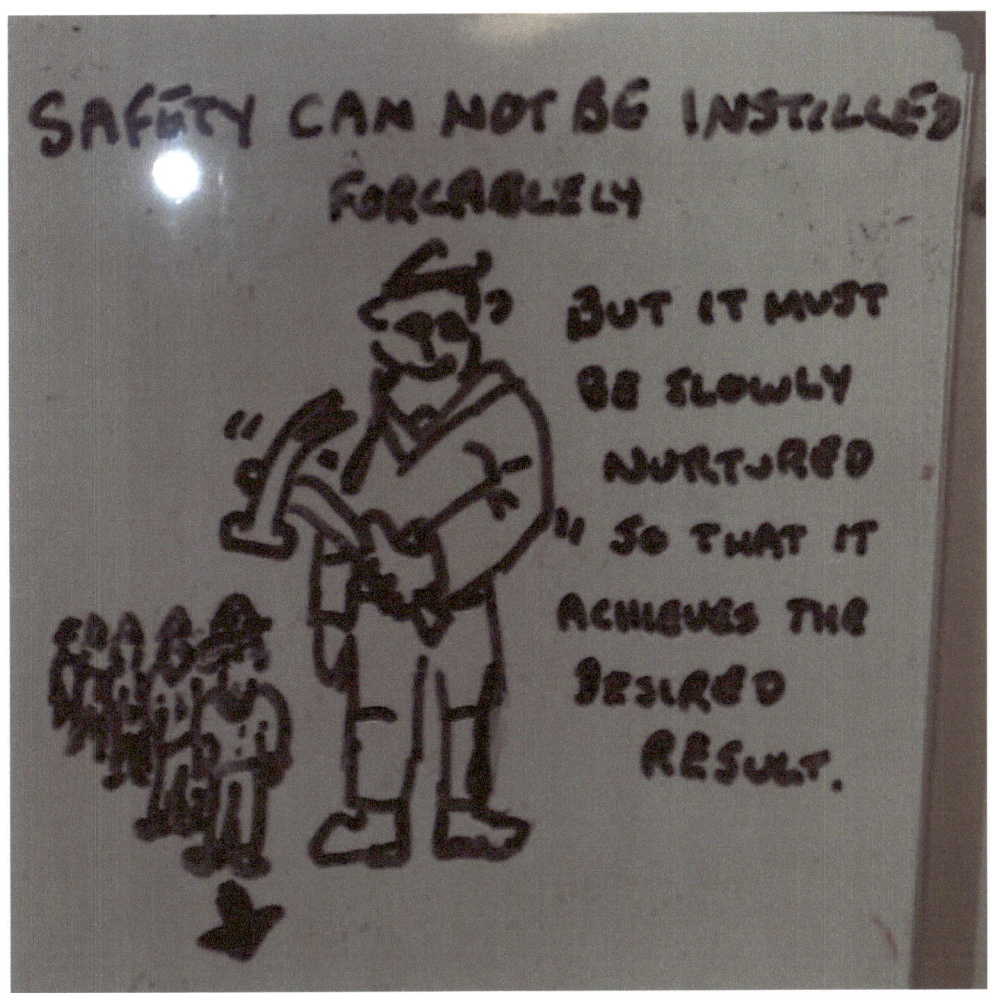

ANY SAFETY REGIME NEEDS TO BE FLEXIBLE IN ITS APPROACH.

IF IT IS HEAVY HANDED AND DRUMMED INTO PEOPLE THEN THEY, LIKE CHILDREN, WILL REBEL AGAINST IT.

I KNOW PEOPLE MAY DISAGREE WITH THIS, BUT JUST THINK BACK TO WHEN WE WERE KIDS.

HOW DID WE REACT TO BEING FORCIBLY TAUGHT?

IF YOU ADOPT A SLOW AND INTERESTING REGIME, THEN YOU HAVE MORE CHANCE OF IT BEING ACCEPTED, USED AND REMEMBERED BY PEOPLE.

REMEMBER: BEING SAFE IS A SLOW PROCESS, BEING UN-SAFE ISN'T.

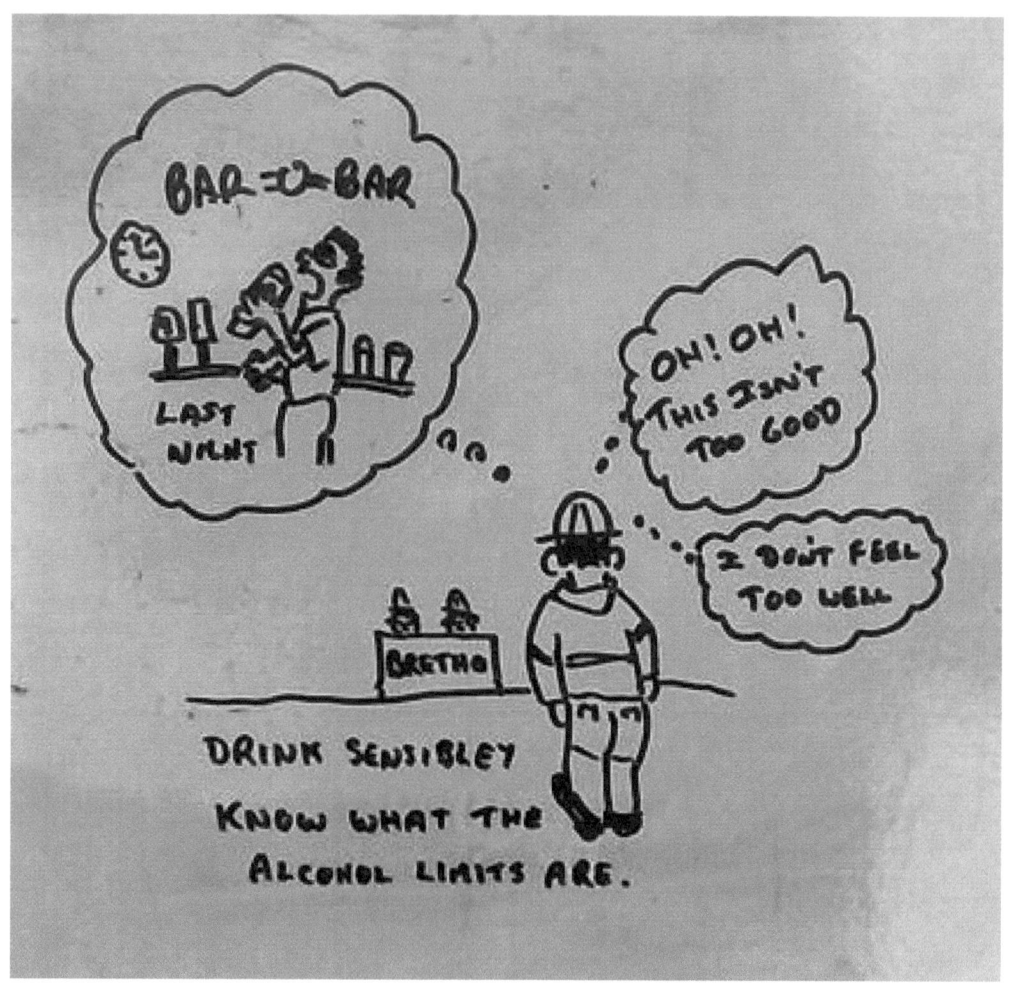

WE ALL KNOW THAT THERE ARE DRINKING LIMITS BOTH AT WORK AND WHEN WE ARE AT HOME.

SOMETIMES WHEN WE ARE IN THAT 'DRINKING MOOD' IT IS SO, SO EASY TO KEEP JUST HAVING ANOTHER ONE, EITHER JUST FOR THE ROAD OR TO PLEASE OUR FRIENDS & BUDDIES.

BUT, STOP, WE MUST BECAUSE IF WE CONTINUE TO DRINK WE RUN THE RISK

OF GETTING CAUGHT EITHER AT WORK OR BY SOME-ONE ELSE.

ALCOHOL CONTINUES TO RISE FOR 4 HOURS AFTER YOU FINISH DRINKING, SO TAKE IT EASY AND DRINK SENSIBLE.

DON'T LOSE YOUR JOB, LISENCE, LIFE OR THAT OF SOME-ONE ELSE'S FOR THE SAKE OF 'JUST 1 MORE'.

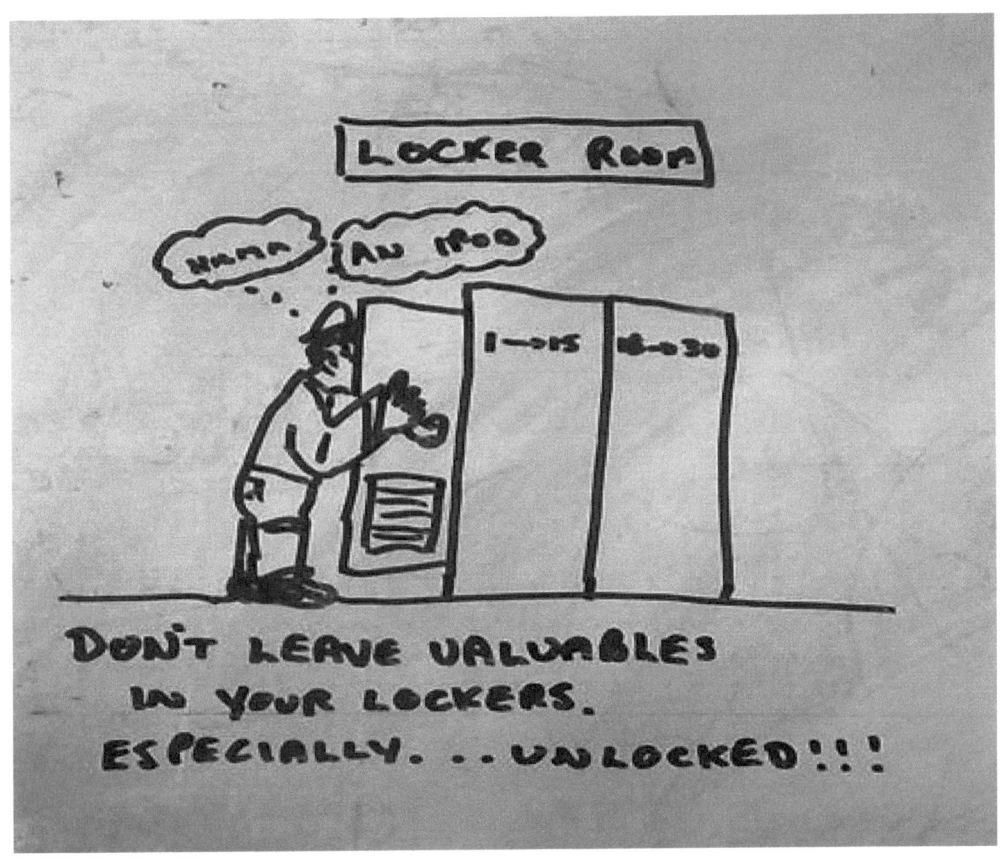

DAY AFTER DAY WE HEAR ABOUT STUFF BEING TAKEN FROM LOCKERS, DESKS, and OFFICES ETC…ETC…ETC.

BUT DO WE LISTEN AND START TO KEEP OUR VALUABLES OR KEEP SAKES LOCKED UP.

NO!

IT'S EITHER TOO MUCH TROUBLE TO DO THAT OR WE ARE JUST PLAIN LAZY.

IN SOCIETY TODAY, I WOULD LOVE TO SAY "THAT YOU CAN TRUST YOUR FELLOW

WORKER OR YOUR FELLOW MAN", BUT UNFORTUNATELY THIS IS NOT THE CASE.

SO, PLEASE KEEP IT SAFE AND STOP SOME-ONE FROM HAVING THATTEMPTATION.IT'S EASIER TO KEEP IT LOCKED THAN TO REPLACE MANY, MANY ITEMS.

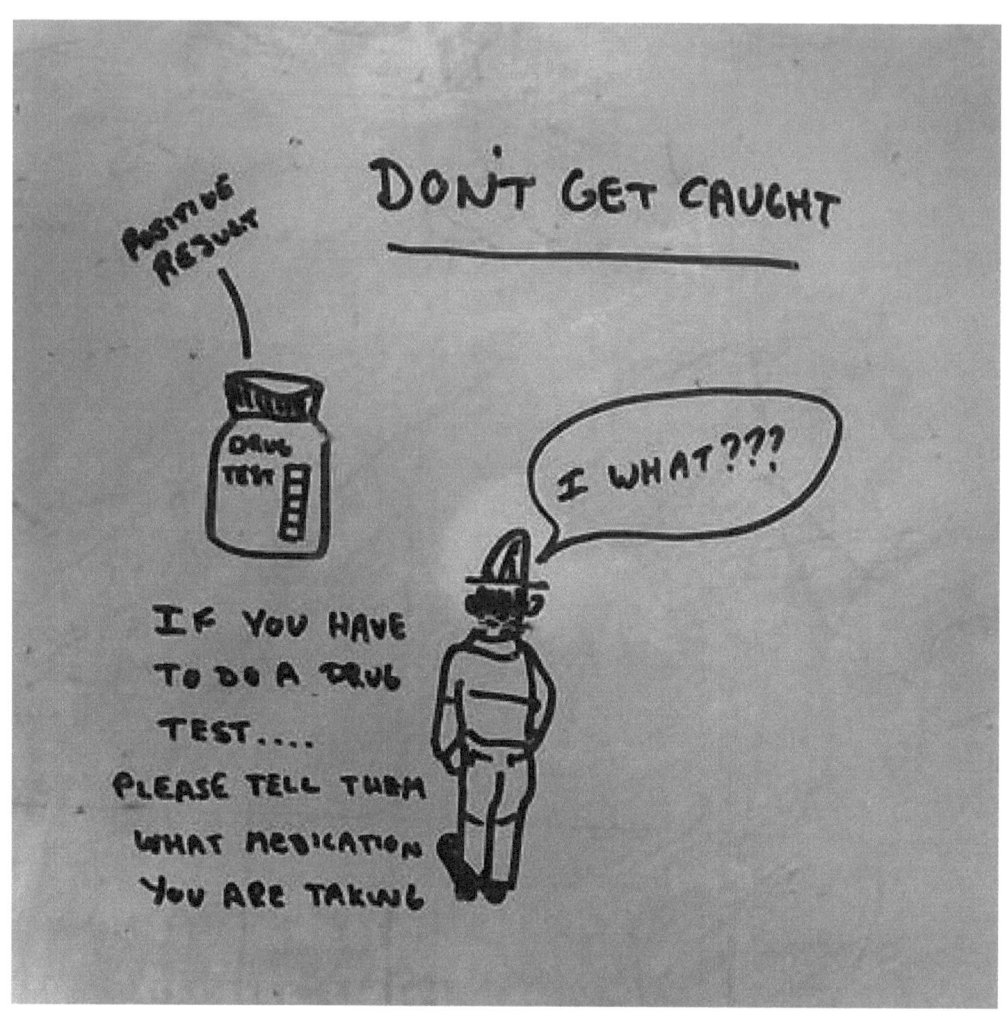

AT WORK YOU MAY HAVE A STRINGENT DRUG AND ALCOHOL POLICY.

WHEN YOU DO HAVE TO DO A DRUG TEST AT WORK, YOU SHOULD ALWAYS TELL THEM WHAT YOU HAVE TAKEN.

WHETHER IT BE PANADOL, NUROFEN, ASPIRIN OR ANY OTHER PRESCRIPTION OR NON-PRESCRIPTION DRUG, IT WILL SHOW UP ON THE SCREENING AND MAY EVEN BE SENT AWAY FOR FURTHER TESTING.

A LOT OF DRUGS THESE DAYS SHARE COMMON INGREDIENTS, SO IT IS BETTER TO LET THEM KNOW FROM THE OUTSET, RATHER THAN GET CAUGHT AND MAYBE LOSE YOUR JOB OVER A LITTLE MIS-UNDERSTANDING.

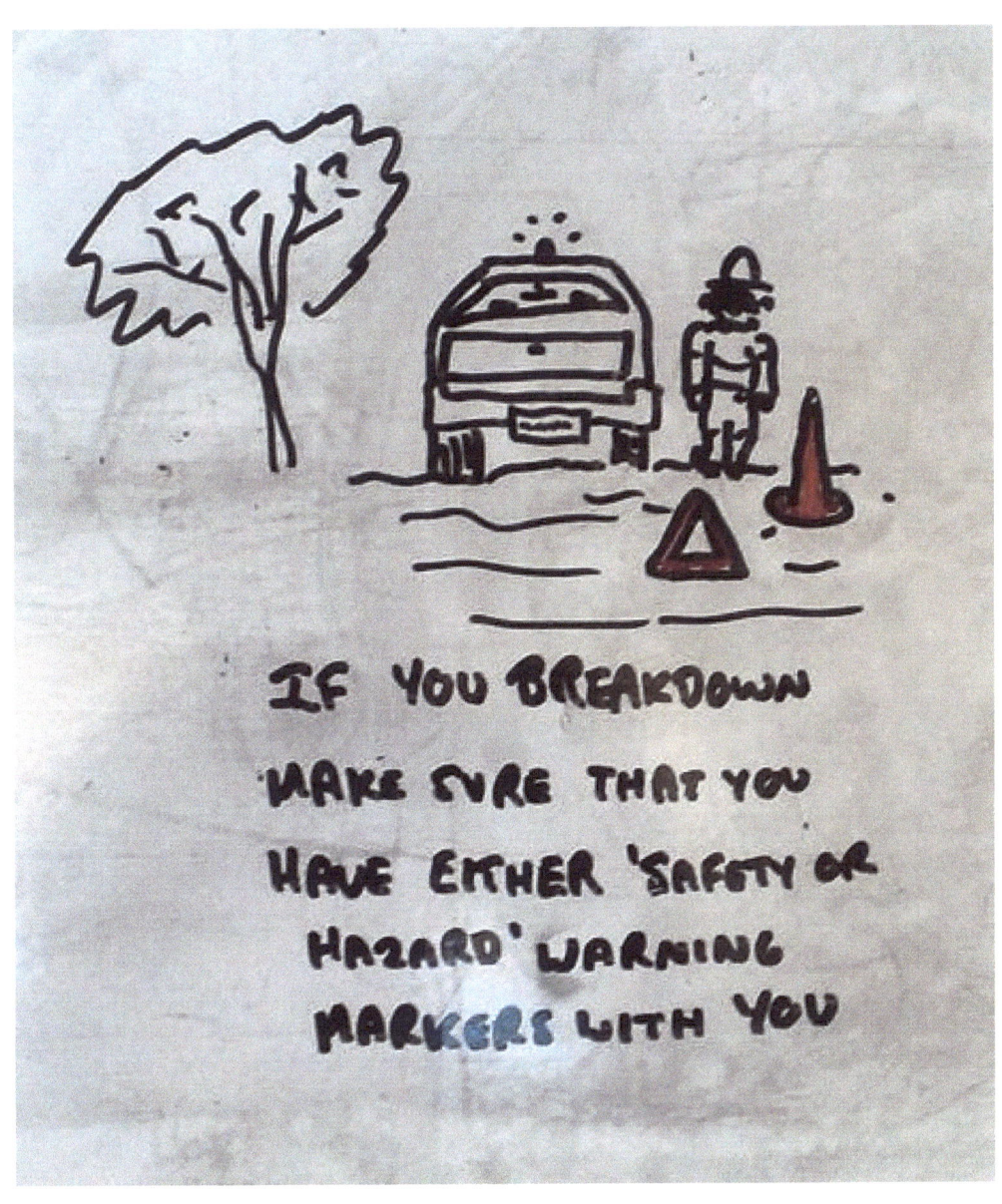

WHEN YOU BREAKDOWN IN YOUR CAR, TRUCK OR WHATEVER VEHICLE YOU ARE DRIVING IT ALWAYS PAYS TO HAVE SOME TYPE OF WARNING OR HAZARD EQUIPMENT WITH YOU.

THIS WAY YOU CAN WARN APPROACHING CARS…ETC THAT YOU HAVE BROKEN DOWN AND THAT THEYNEED TO SLOW DOWN WHEN THEY PASS OR GO AROUND YOU.

IT'S BETTER TO BE SEEN, THAN TO HAVE SOME-ONE NOT SEE YOU AND BE THE CAUSE OF ANOTHER ACCIDENT.

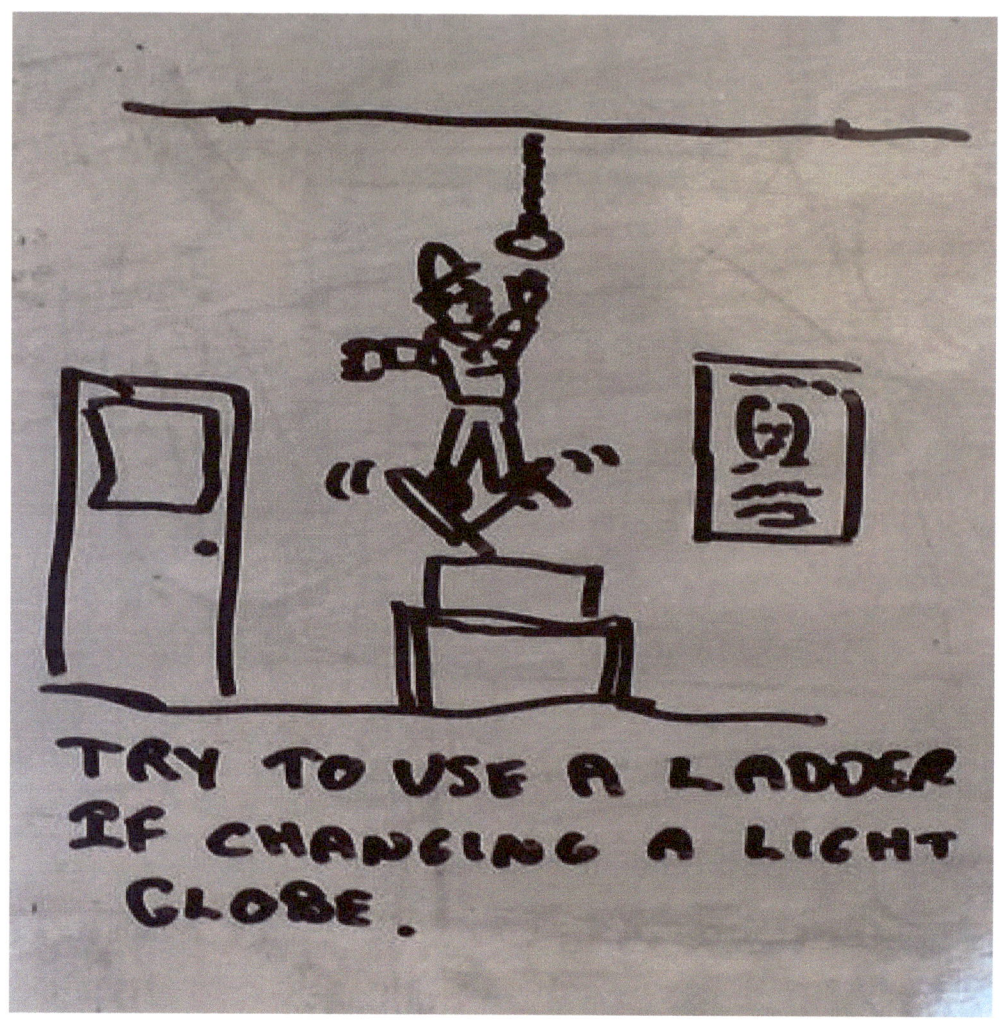

"SEEM FAMILIAR?"

WHEN WE DON'T HAVE A LADDER TO REACH FOR THINGS, WHETHER IT BE FROM CHANGING LIGHT GLOBES TO THAT ALL ALLUSIVE BOX OF KEEPSAKES, HIDDEN AT THE BACK OF A WARDROBE; HOW OFTEN HAVE WE STOOD ON RICKETY OLD CHAIRS OR MILK CRATES TO REACH FOR THEM?

EVERYONE OF US HAS DONE IT AT SOME STAGE IN OUR LIVES, YET WE STILL CONTINUE TO DO IT AT TIMES.

IT'S JUST A SHAME THAT WE DON'T PRACTISE BEING SAFE WHEN WE DO IT. IT'S ABOUT TIME WE THOUGHT AHEAD TO WHAT COULD HAPPEN AND JUST GET A LADDER OR A SET OF SMALL STEPS.

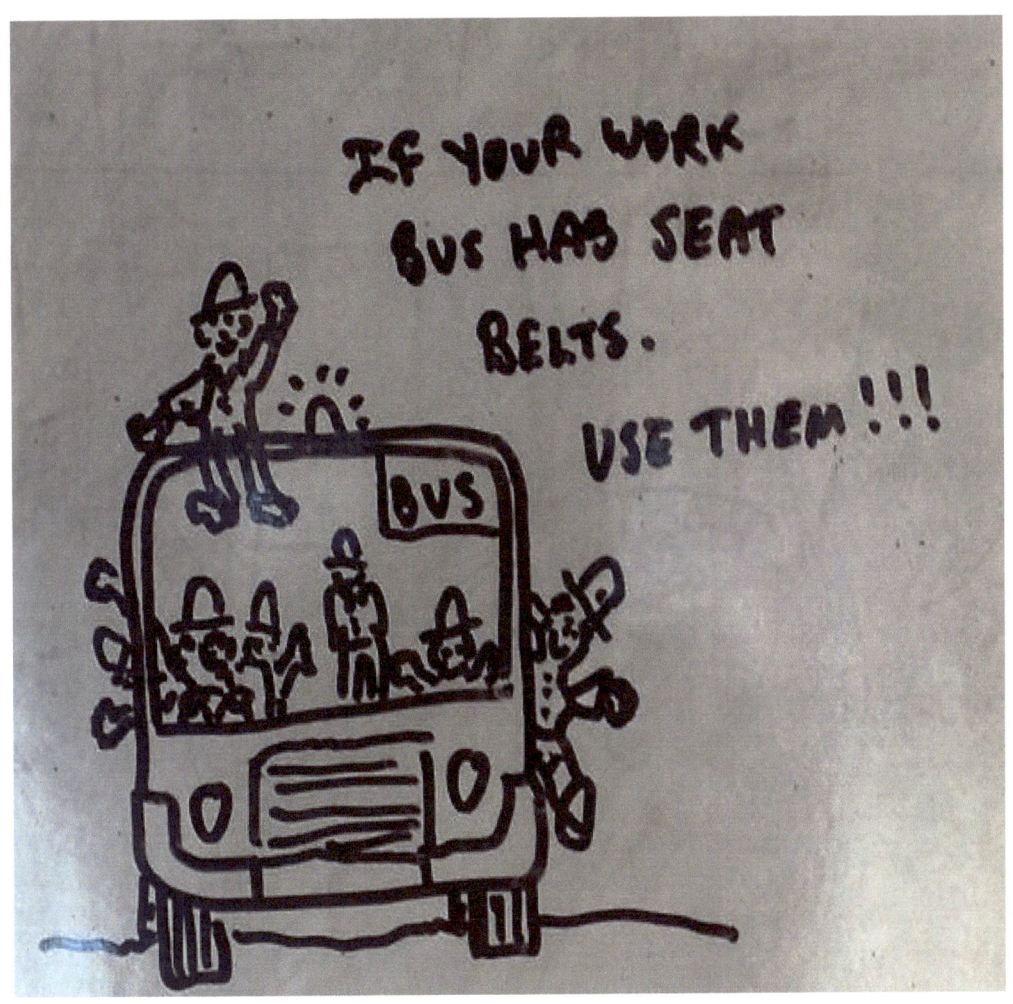

AGAIN WE HAVE YET ANOTHER ROAD SAFETY MESSAGE. IT'S STILL THE SAME.

BELT UP TO SAVE LIVES.

MANY BUSES, PUBLIC TRANSPORT OR EVEN WORK PLACE PEOPLE MOVERS

HAVE SEAT BELTS IN THEM.

THEY ARE THERE FOR A REASON AND WE NEED TO USE THEM.

DON'T LET PEER PRESSURE OR JUST BEING 'ONE OF THE LADS' STOP YOU FROM DOING THE RIGHT THING.

BELT UP AND SAVE YOUR LIFE & MAKE SURE THAT THOSE AROUND YOU DO THE SELF SAME THING.

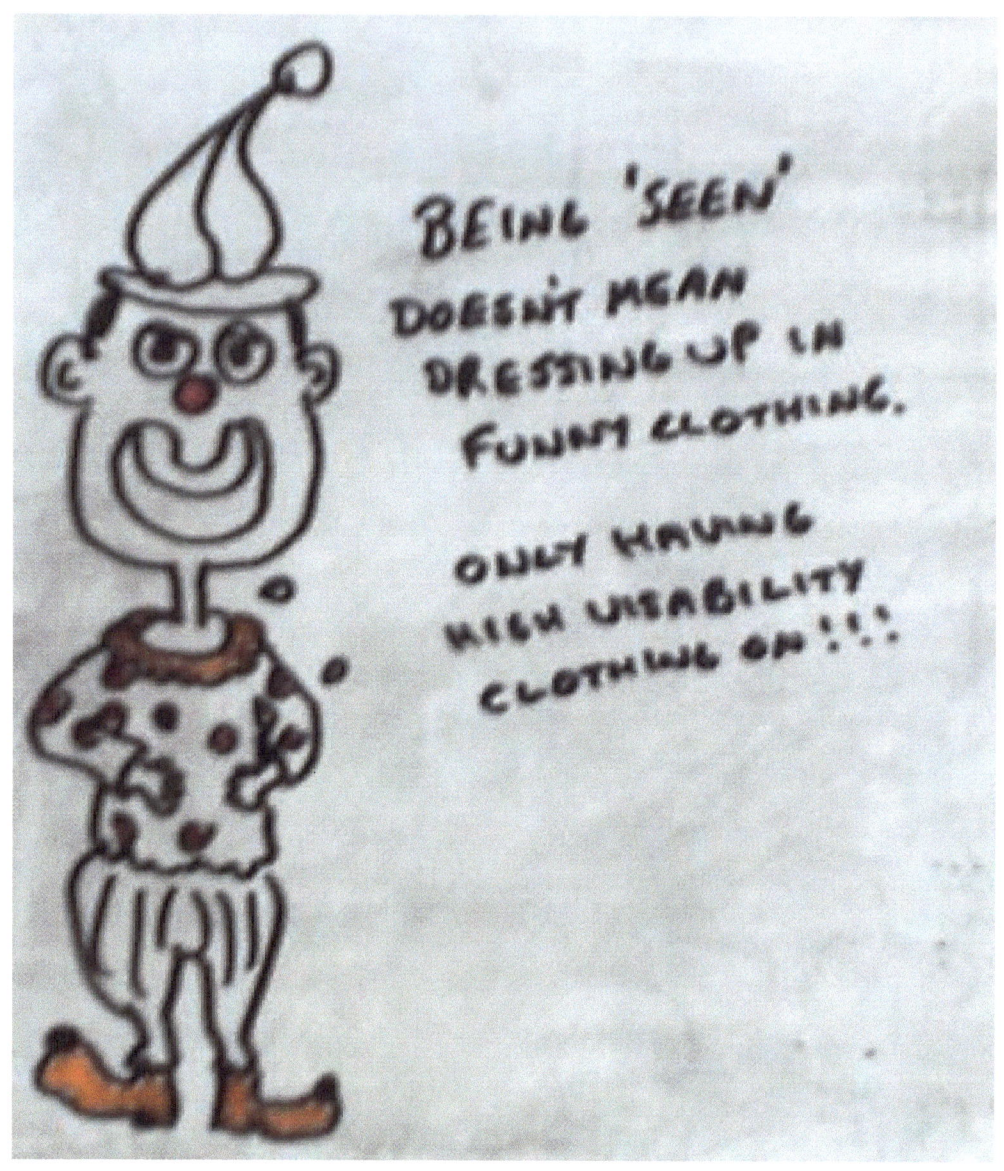

MOST WORK PLACES THESE DAYS REQUIRE THAT YOU WEAR 'HIGH VISIBILITY' CLOTHING.

THIS IS BECAUSE THEY WANT YOU TO BE SEEN BY APPROACHING DRIVERSEITHER IN CARS, WORK TRUCKS OR JUST SO THAT YOU CAN BE SEEN BY OTHER PEOPLE.

WHEN WORKING AT NIGHT, THE HIGH VISIBILITY CLOTHING SHOULD INCLUDE REFLECTIVE STRIPES, SO THAT THEY WILL REFLECT LIGHTS FROM APPROACHING VEHICLES.

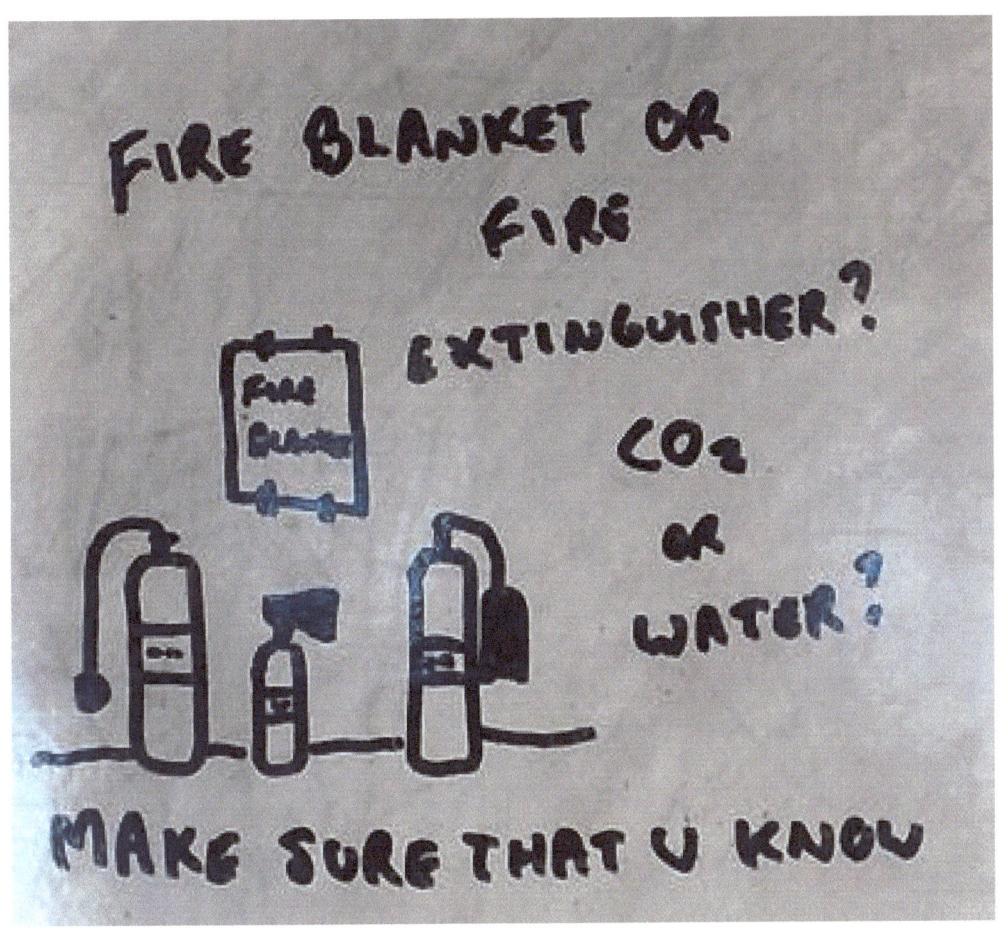

USING THE RIGHT FIRE EXTINGUISHER OR FIRE PREVENTION METHOD IS VERY IMPORTANT.

IF WE USE THE WRONG ONE, THEN WE RUN THE RISK OF THE FIRE SPREADING, BEING INJURED OURSELVES OR CAUSING INJURY TO OTHERS.

CO2, WATER, FOAM, FIRE BLANKET ETC, ARE ALL DIFFERENT TYPES OF EXTINGUISHERS OR EQUIPMENT THAT WE CAN USE, BUT WE HAVE TO LEARN WHICH ONE IS THE RIGHT ONE FOR ANY GIVEN SITUATION.

IF YOU ARE UN-SURE THEN YOU SHOULD ASK YOUR SUPERVISORS, MANAGERS OR YOUR OH&S DEPARTMENTS ABOUT WHICH ONE TO USE.

DOING THIS DOES NOT MAKE YOU LOOK SILLY OR ANYTHING ELSE, BUT DEMONSTRATES A SINCERE DESIRE TO 'KNOW & LEARN'.

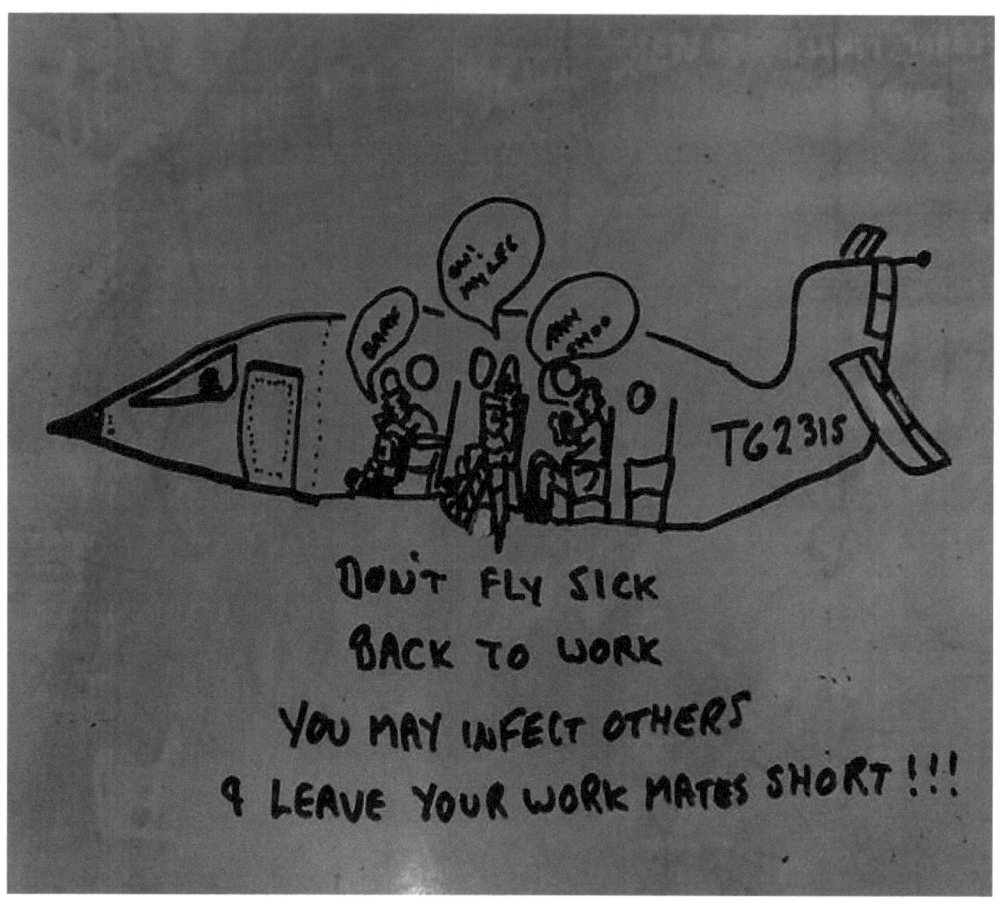

PEOPLE TEND TO THINK THAT THEY ARE INDISPENSIBLE AT WORK AND SO THEY WILL ALWAYS GO TO WORK, COME HELL OR HIGH WATER.

IT DOESN'T MATTER IF THEY HAVE A COLD, MUSCLE STRAINS, A FEVER AND/OR A MYRIAD OF OTHER AILMENTS.

NOT ONLY DO WE RUN THE RISK OF MAKING WHAT WE HAVE WORSE, BUT WE CAN PASS IT ON TO OTHER PEOPLE WHICH IN TURN MAY MEAN THEY MAY HAVE TO HAVE TIME OFF OR THEY IN TURN MAY INFECT SOME-ONE ELSE, PARTICULARLY ANOTHER FAMILY MEMBER.

SO DON'T TRAVEL SICK AND DON'T GO TO WORK.

STAY HOME, GET WELL AND JUST GET BETTER.

YOUR HEALTH IS IMPORTANT AND YOUR WORK WILL ALWAYS BE THERE.

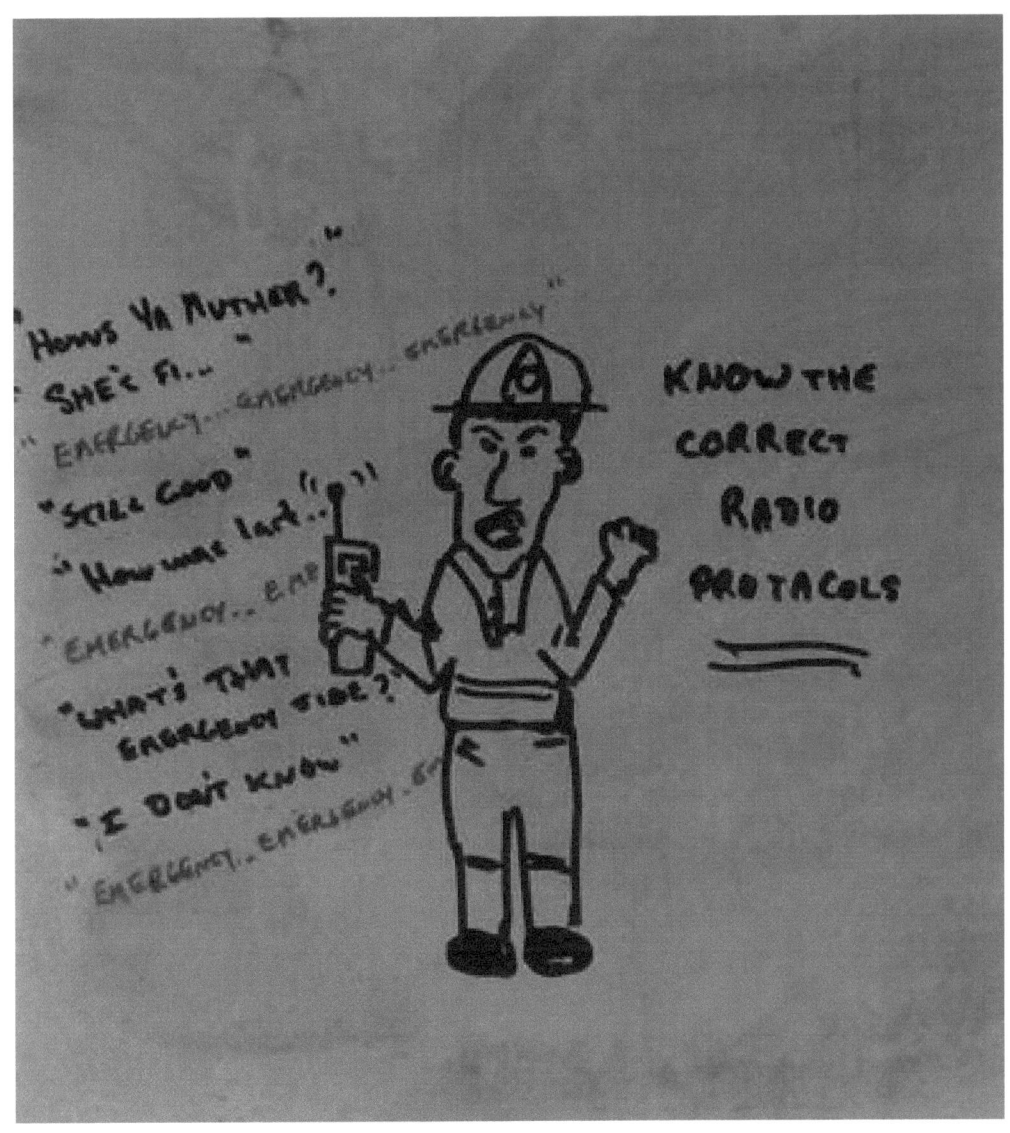

ON MINE SITES AND OTHER WORK PLACES YOU MAY HAVE NEED TO USE UHF OR VHF RADIOS.

IF YOU DO, THEN YOU HAVE TO ADHERE TO ANY RULES PERTAINING TO THEM AND THERE USE.

IF THERE IS AN EMERGENCY, YOU WILL FIND THAT RADIO CHATTER SHOULD STOP COMPLETELY UNLESS YOU HAVE TO NOTIFY OTHERS THAT YOU ARE APPROACHING A CERTAIN AREA.

SO USE COMMON SENSE AND HAVE RESPECT FOR OTHER RADIO USERS.

DON'T STOP SOME-ONE GETTING THE HELP THAT THEY NEED.

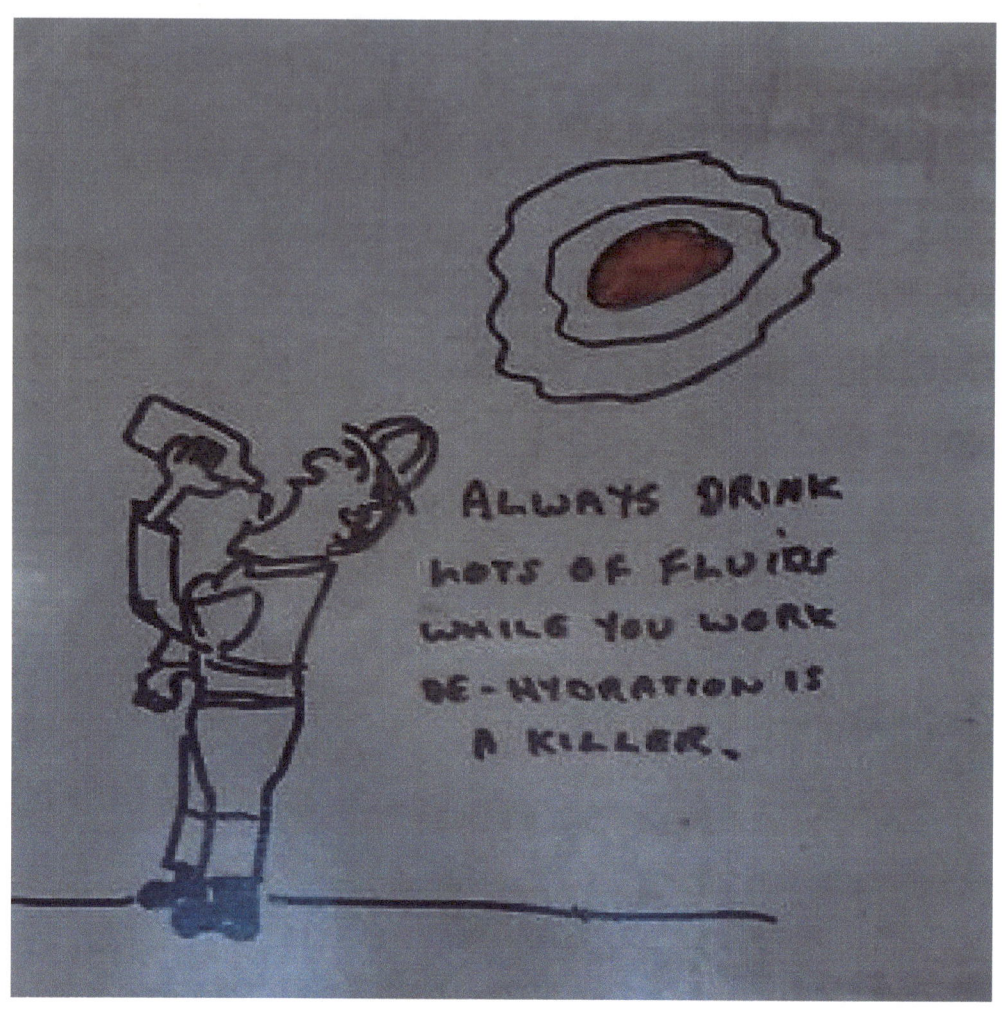

IN AUSTRALIA AND OTHER HOT AND HUMID COUNTRIES YOU WILL NEED TO KEEP YOUR FLUIDS UP.

THAT IS, YOU SHOULD DRINK LOTS OF WATER SO THAT YOU DO NOT DEHYDRATE AND DIE.

IN MOST CASES BY THE TIME YOU REALIZE THAT YOU ARE THIRSTY AND YOUR MOUTH IS DRY, THAT YOU ARE ALREADY DEHYDRATED.

YOU SHOULD DRINK WHEN YOU ARE NOT THIRSTY, TO START WITH.

THAT WAY YOUR BODY WILL ABSORB THE FLUIDS TO START WITH AND THEN ALL YOU NEED TO DO, IS TOP IT UP AS YOU WORK DURING THE DAY OR NIGHT

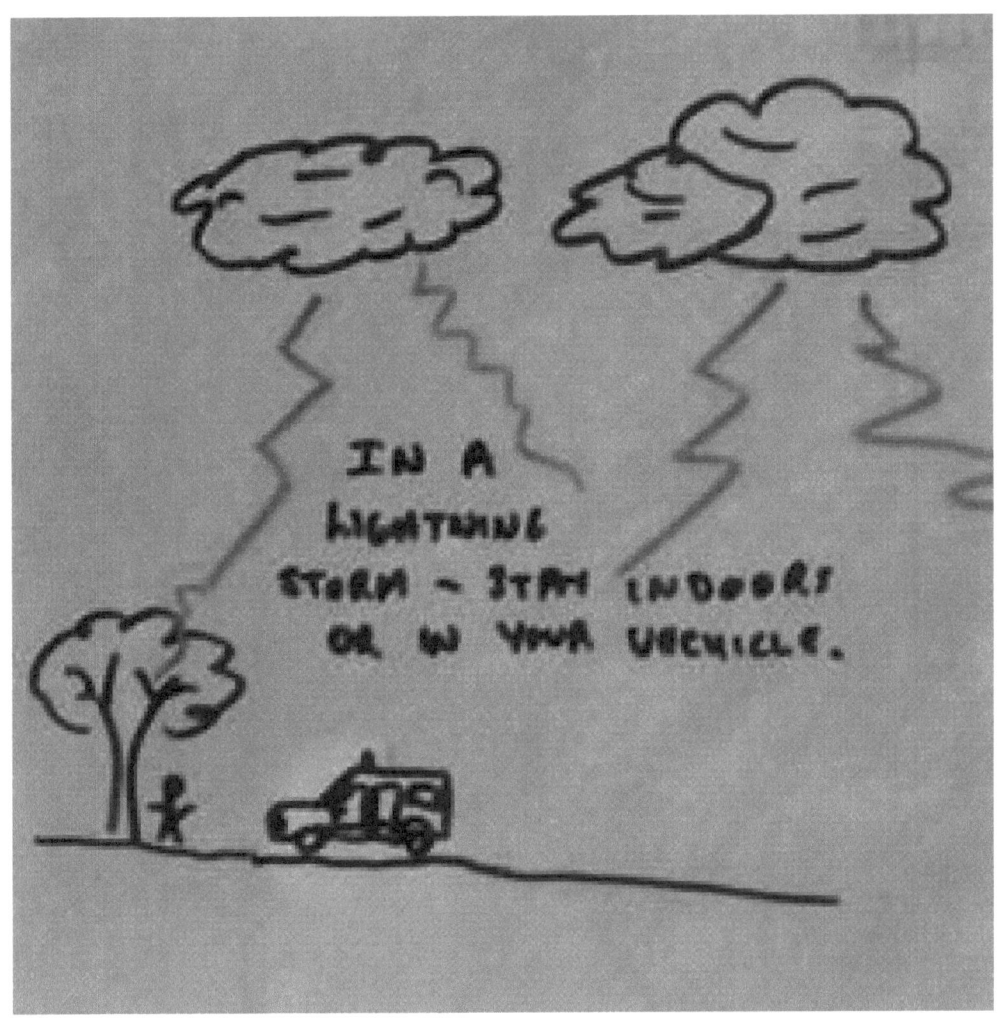

BEING OUT IN A STORM IS CERTAINLY NOT IDEAL, UNLESS OF COURSE YOU ARE A STORM CHASER OR A PHOTOGRAPHER.

IF YOU ARE OUT IN ONE YOU SHOULD STAY IN YOUR VEHICLE WITH THE WINDOWS UP OR YOU SHOULD FIND SHELTER INSIDE A BUILDING. YOU SHOULD NEVER STAND UNDER A TREE, SEEK HIGH GROUND, OR HAVE METAL NEAR OR ON YOUR BODY.

DO NOT USE A PHONE AS THIS CAN ALSO ATTRACT LIGHTNING.

IF YOU HEAR A WARNING OVER YOUR RADIO TO FINISH WHAT YOU ARE DOING AND GET UNDER COVER, THEN YOU SHOULD DO IT POSTE HASTE.

LIGHTNING CAN KILL AND IT CAN LEAVE SEVERE WOUNDS.

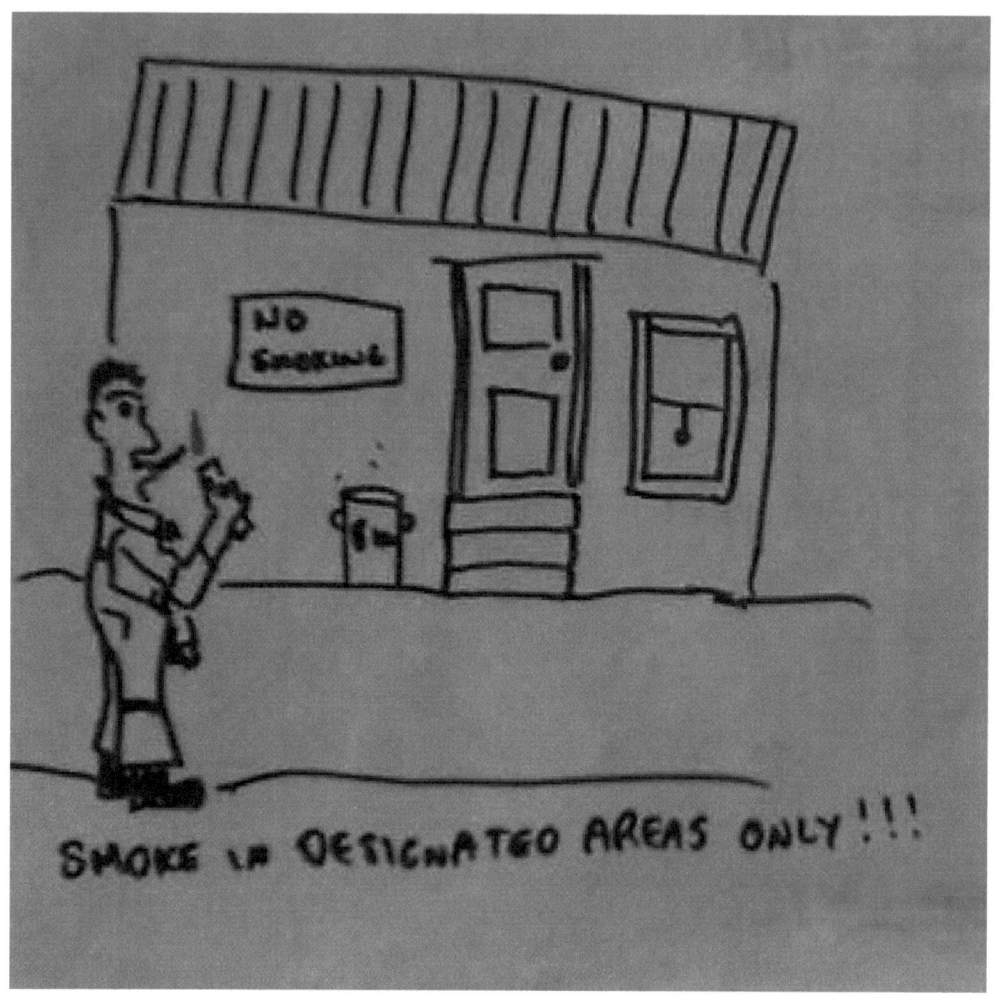

IN MANY COUNTRIES AROUND THE WORLD SMOKING IN CERTAIN AREAS HAS BEEN INSTITUTED.

THIS IS TO SAVE PEOPLE FROM INHALING SMOKE FROM THOSE WHO LIKE TO LIGHT UP AND HAVE A CIGARETTE.

IT'S CALLED 'PASSIVE SMOKING' AND WITHOUT A DOUBT, MANY, IF NOT ALL OF YOU WOULD HAVE HEARD ABOUT IT ALREADY.

SO IF YOU SEE A SIGN SAYING "NO SMOKING" YOU SHOULD ADHERE TO IT AND FIND A PLACE THAT ADVERTISES THAT "YOU CAN SMOKE HERE."

SOMETIMES IT CAN BE AN IMPOSITION, BUT WE MUST ALL OBEY THE SIGNS, OTHERWISE WE RUN THE RISK OF FINES OR HAVING OUR MANAGER TALK TO US.

LIGHT UP OR BUTT OUT…IT'S YOUR CHOICE.

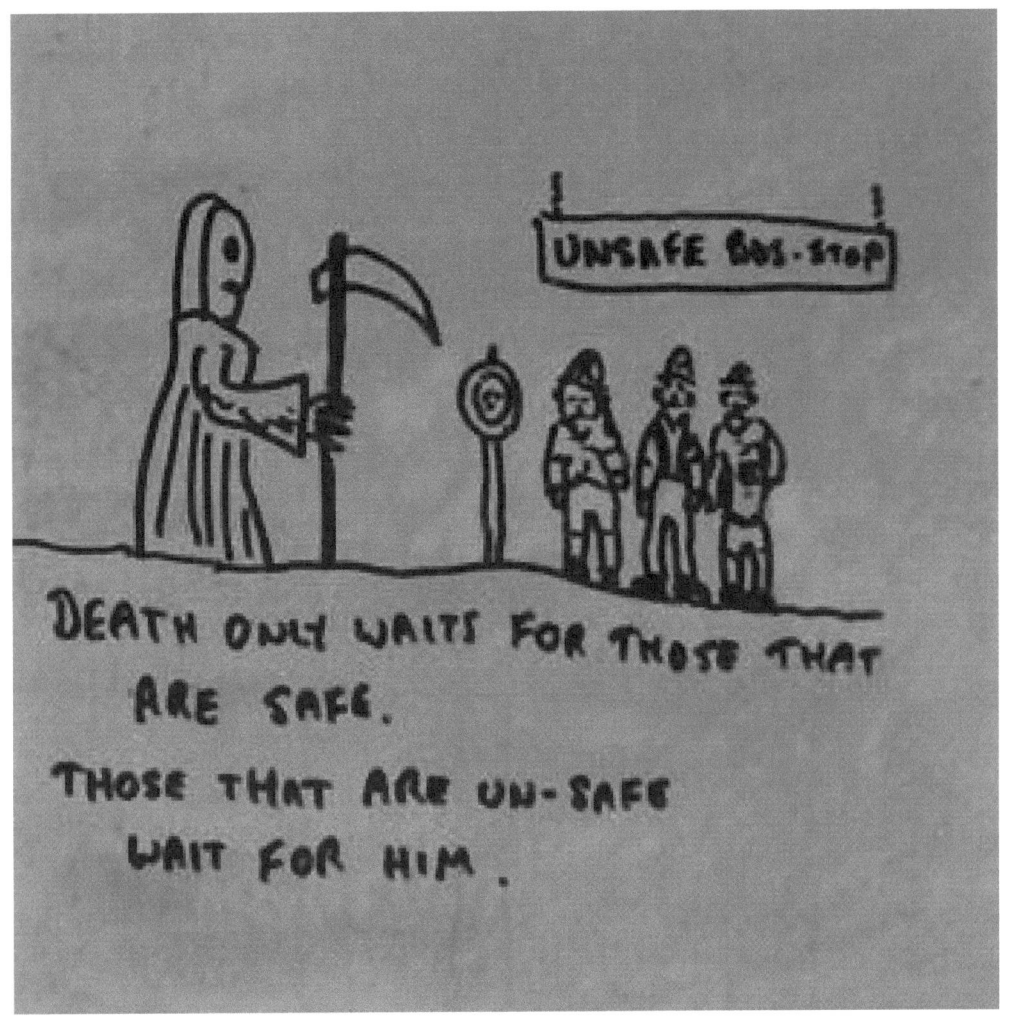

LIGHT HEARTED DRAWINGS ARE FUN, BUT THEY ALSO CONVEY A MESSAGE.

DEATH DOES WAIT FOR THOSE THAT PLAY AND WORK SAFE, BECAUSE THEY REALIZE WHAT THE CONSEQUENCES ARE IF THEY DON'T.

IT'S THE PEOPLE THAT TAKE SHORT CUTS; DON'T KNOW THE PROPER WAY OR A MYRIAD OF OTHER WAYS TO BE UNSAFE THAT WAIT AROUND FOR DEATH TO SHOW UP.

OF COURSE IT MAY NOT BE DEATH, BUT SOME FORM OF DIS-ABILITY THAT HAPPENS TO THEM OR TO OTHERS.

SO, UN-SAFE…IT'S NOT THE WAY I WANT TO GO.

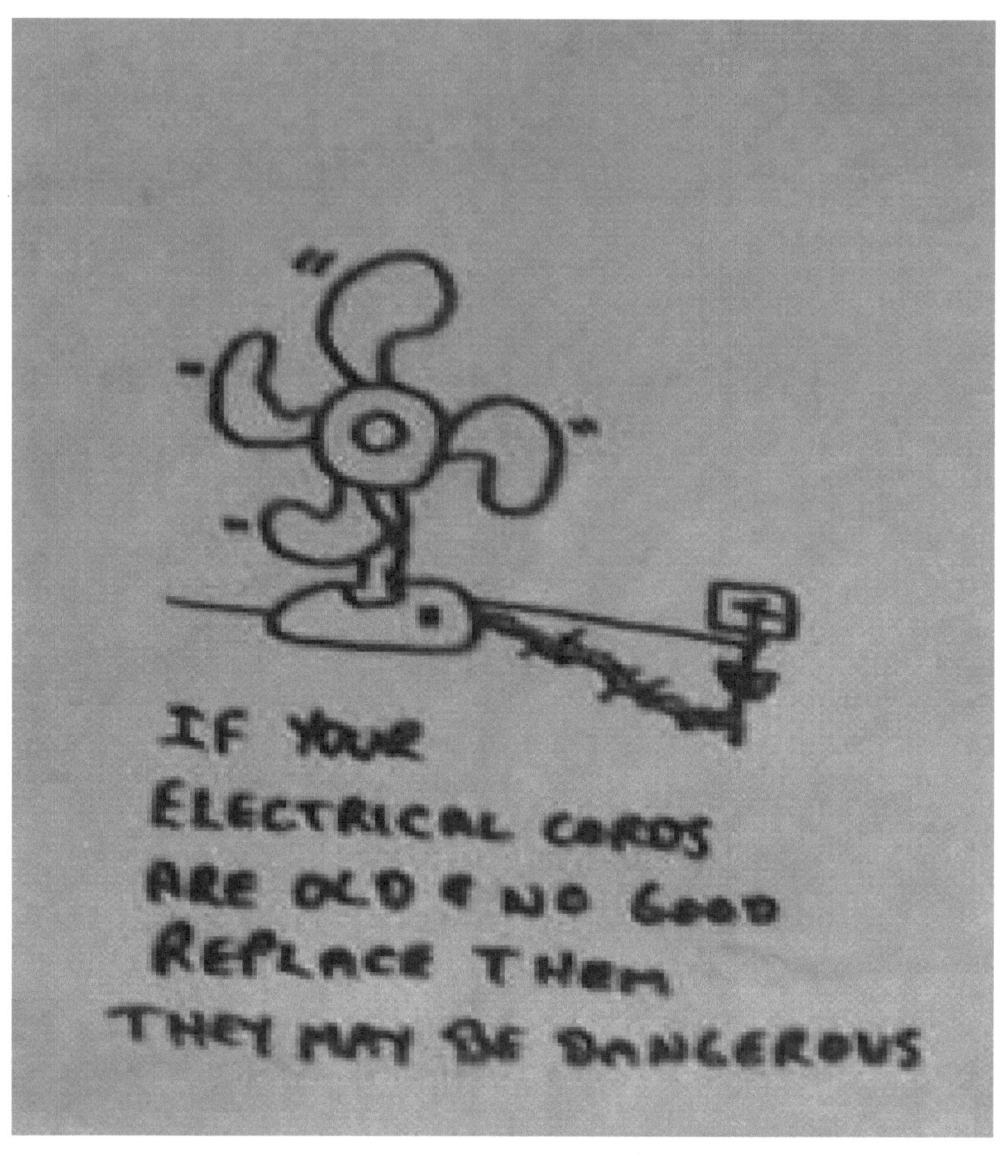

MANY MINES AND WORK PLACES HAVE PERIODICAL CHECKS OF THEIR ELECTRICAL EQUIPMENT AND YOU SHOULD ALSO DO THE SAME AT HOME.

IF THE CORD IS FRAYED AND OLD, IT MAY BE A 'DEATH TRAP' WAITING TO HAPPEN.

THEY CAN CAUSE INJURY, DEATH AND MAY EVEN BLOW ALL THE FUSES OUT &TRIP THE POWER.

WHICH YOU MAY KNOW CAN CAUSE DAMAGE TO OTHER EQUIPMENT.

SO ALWAYS CHECK FOR FRAYED CORDS AND THAT ALL ELECTRICAL EQUIPMENT WORKS ON A REGULAR BASIS.

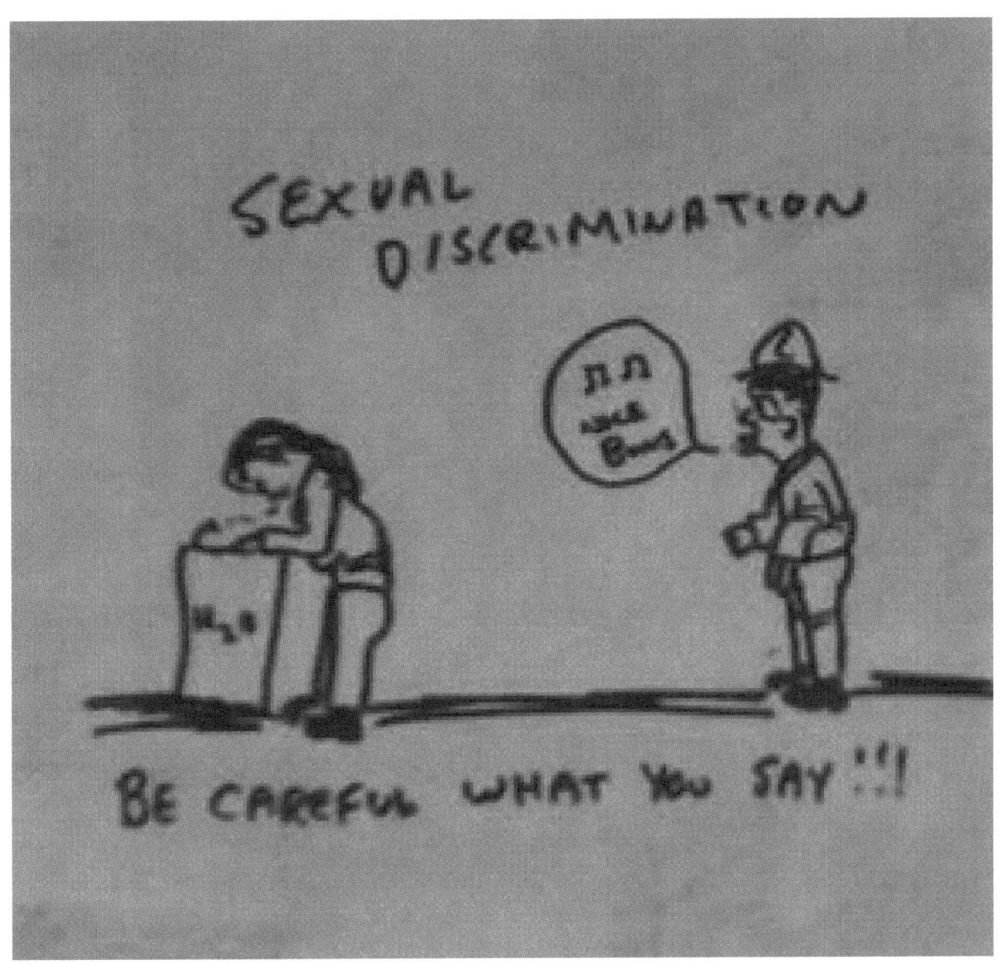

WHAT A MINEFIELD THIS IS!

WHAT WE USED TO CONSIDER AS PERFECT NORMAL BEHAVIOUR WHICH INCLUDED WHISTLING, OGLING, MAKING RUDE AND UNSAVOURY REMARKS IS NOW A THING OF THE PAST.

HOPEFULLY IT IS ANYWAY.

BETWEEN FRIENDS YOU CAN HAVE THE ODD WHISTLE OR LAUGH, BUT WHEN YOU CARRY IT INTO THE EXTREME AND START DOING IT TO OTHER PEOPLE OR JUST PERSIST WITH IT, THEN IT CAN BECOME A CASE OF SEXUAL DISCRIMINATION OR JUST PLAIN OLD DISCRIMINATION.

IT DOES NOT MATTER IF YOU ARE FEMALE OR EVEN MALE.

SO CURB THE URGE AND ACT WITH RESPECT TOWARDS OTHERS.

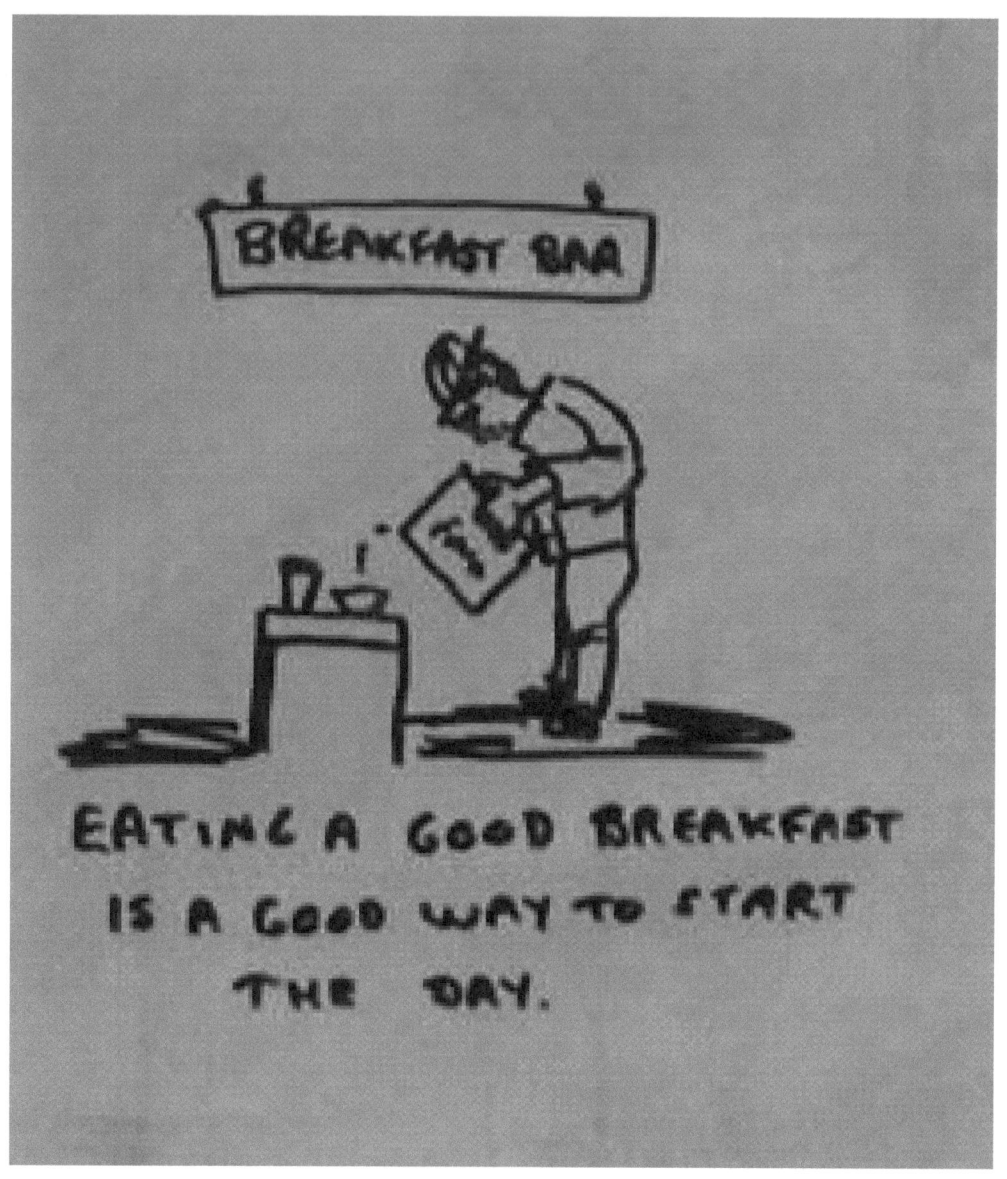

MANY PEOPLE WILL KNOW THIS ONE, ALREADY.

A GOOD WAY TO START ANY DAY OR NIGHTSHIFT IS WITH A GOOD HEARTY, AND YES, MAYBE HEALTHY MEAL.

THAT WAY YOU WILL HAVE MORE ENERGY DURING THE DAY OR DURING YOUR SHIFT UNTIL YOU CAN HAVE ANOTHER BREAK TO FILL UP AGAIN.

IT ALSO CAN PROMOTE GOOD RESPONSE TIMES, CLEAR THINKING AND PROVIDE   YOU WITH ENERGY.

EAT WISE…EAT HEALTHY…EAT TO SURVIVE

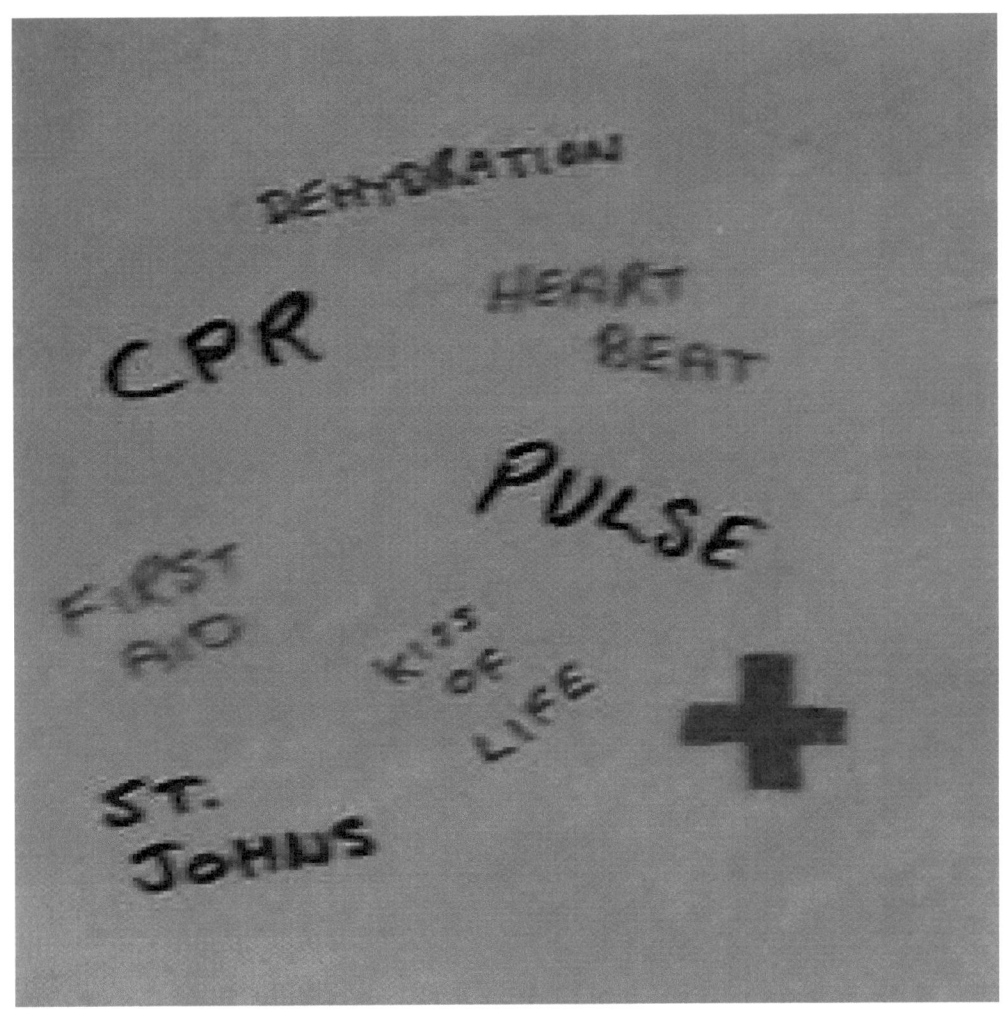

HOW MANY OF US KNOW FIRST AID?

IN MANY OCCUPATIONS IT IS NOW PART OF THE WORK REQUIREMENTS THAT YOU POSSESS A FIRST AID CERTIFICATE.

IT ALSO PAYS TO DO A FIRST AID COURSE EVEN IF YOU DON'T NEED ONE FOR WORK, BECAUSE THERE MAY OME A TIME WHERE YOU ATTEND AN ACCIDENT   AND YOU MAY NEED TO RENDER ASSISTANCE TO SAVE SOME-ONE.

IT'S NOT AS DAUNTING AS IT SOUNDS.

BEING ABLE TO LOOK AFTER SOME-ONE WHO NEEDS HELP IS WHAT MAKES US UNIQUE. IT SHOWS THAT WE DO CARE.

SO…DO YOU CARE ENOUGH TO DO IT?

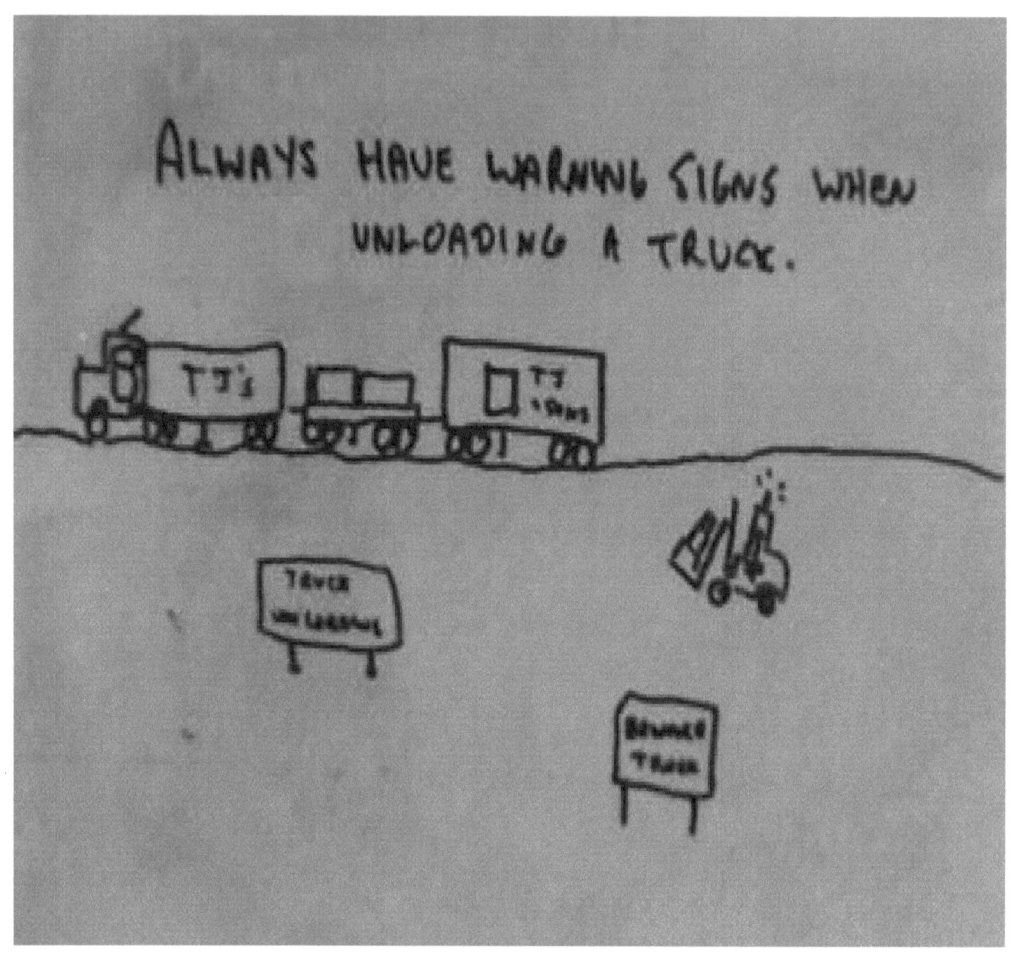

IN MANY WORK PLACES WHEN A TRUCK IS EITHER BEING LOADED OR UNLOADED THEY HAVE SIGNS WARNING APPROACHING PEOPLE THAT THE AREA IS HAZARDOUS AND TO BE CAREFUL.

EVEN WITH SIGNS ERECTED, PEOPLE STILL COME CLOSE TO THE TRUCK OR FORKLIFT ETC WITHOUT MUCH THOUGHT FOR THE CONSEQUENCES.

SO KEEP AN EYE OUT.

IF YOU KNOW THAT AN AREA IS UN-SAFE BECAUSE THEY ARE MOVING PALLETS OR GOODS AROUND TAKE CARE AND GIVE THEM A WIDE BERTH.

SEE THE SIGNS & BEWARE THE SIGNS

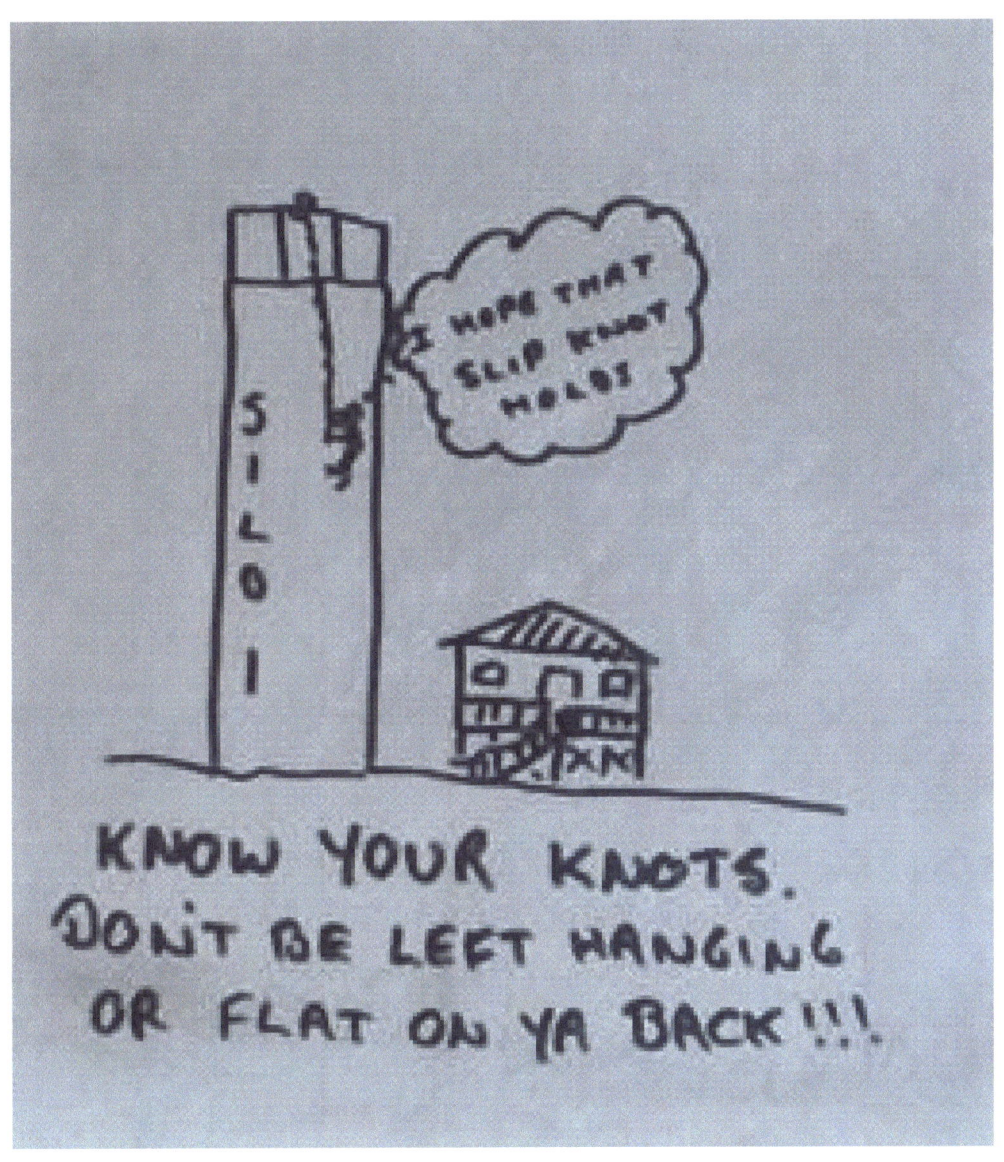

WHEN YOU WORK IN A VARIETY OF JOBS, YOU MAY NEED TO KNOW SOME DIFFERENT TYPES OF KNOTS.

WHETHER YOU ARE A TRUCK DRIVER, IN MINES RESCUE, OR JUST TYING DOWN A LOAD ON THE BACK OF A TRAILER, YOU MAY HAVE TO KNOW HOW TO DO IT   CORRECTLY.

THERE IS NOTHING WORSE THAN HAVING A LOAD COME UNDONE ON A ROAD OR IF YOUR LIFE DEPENDS ON IT.

SO IF YOU NEED TO TIE SOMETHING DOWN OR ABSAIL DOWN A SILO ETC, KNOW YOUR KNOTS.

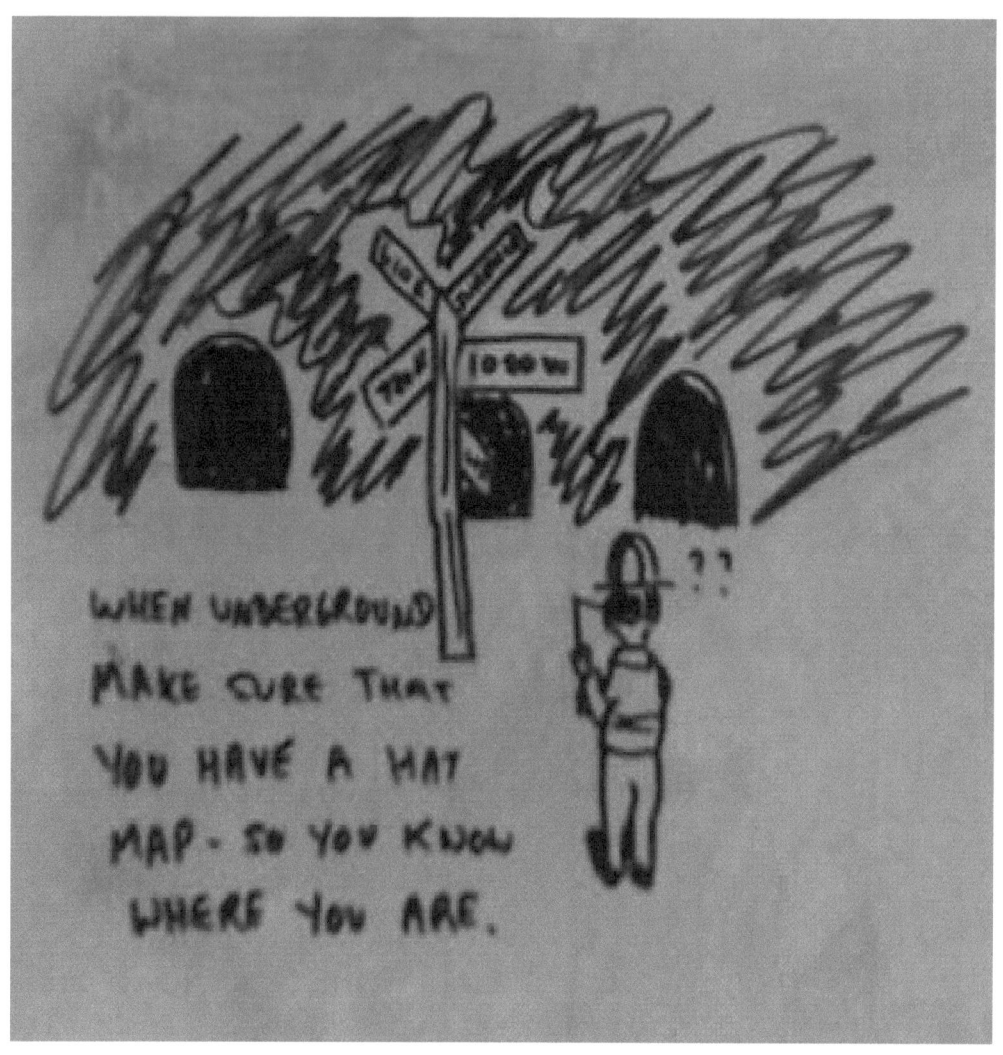

WORKING IN UNDERGROUND MINES, THEY HAVE LITTLE THINGS CALLED 'HAT MAPS'.

THESE ARE HANDY LITTLE MAPS THAT YOU STOW UNDER YOUR HAT OR IN A POCKET SOMEWHERE.

THEY SHOW YOU A ROUGH LAYOUT OF THE MINE WITH ROUTES, ESCAPE WAYSETC SO THAT YOU KNOW WHERE YOU ARE GOING.

IF YOURS IS OUT OF DATE YOU SHOULD ASK FOR AN UPDATED ONE.

IT CAN SAVE TIME & SAVE LIFES. SO MAKE SURE YOU HAVE YOURS.

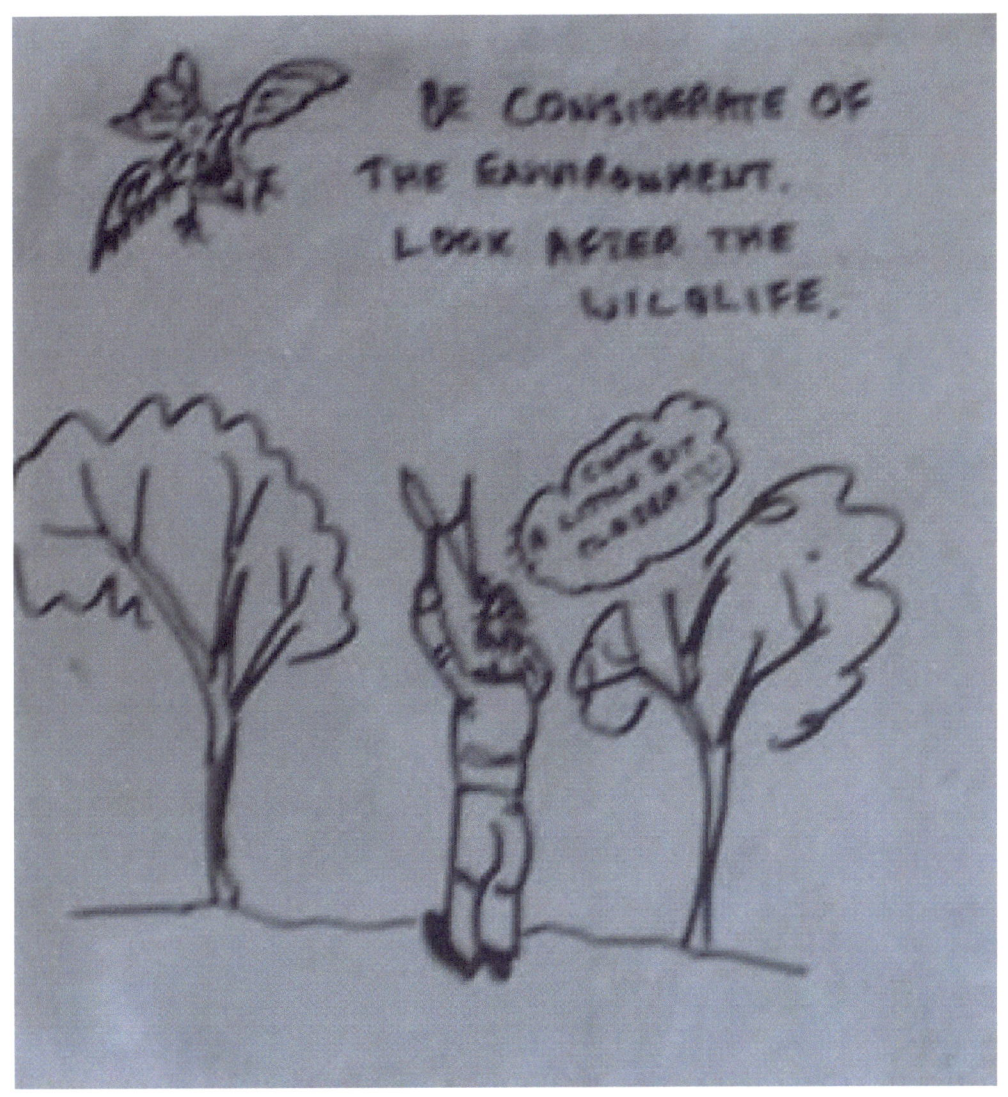

PEOPLE TREAT THE ENVIRONMENT AND THE ANIMALS IN IT BADLY.

WE SEEM TO TAKE PLEASURE IN WATCHING SOME ANIMALS SUFFER, NOMATTER WHAT THEY ARE.

I BELIEVE THAT NO MATTER WHAT TYPE OF ANIMAL IT IS, WE SHOULD TREAT IT WITH RESPECT AND NOT SUBMIT IT TO CRUELTY.

MANY ANIMALS ARE DISAPPEARING AROUND US NOW, WITHOUT US ADDING TO   THE CARNAGE THAT THEY ALREADY SUFFER.

ANIMALS ARE THERE TO MAKE US REMEMBER:

THAT WE WERE ALL ANIMALS, ONCE.

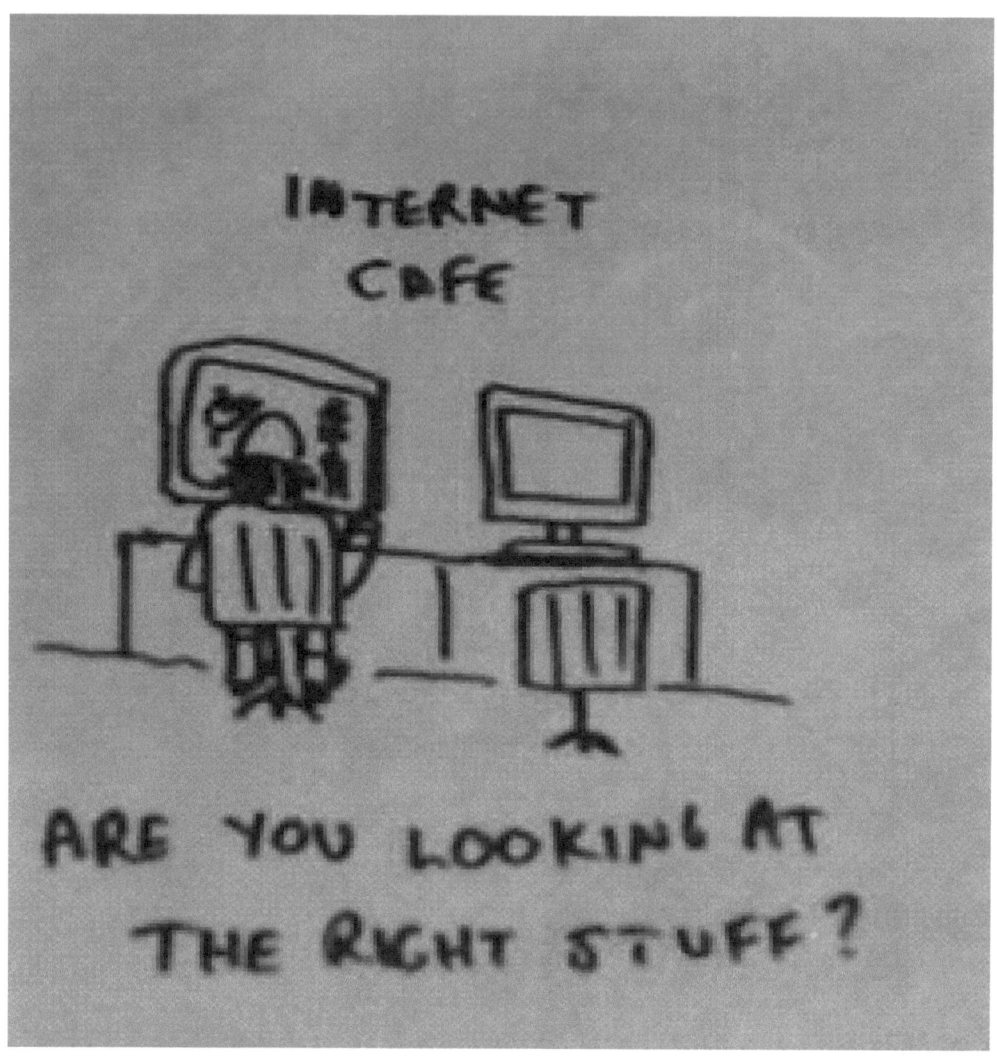

MANY WORK PLACES HAVE COMPUTERS THESE DAYS, EITHER ON YOUR OWN DESK, SOME-ONE ELSE'S OR IN AN 'INTERNET CAFÉ'.

MOST COMPANIES HAVE RULES ABOUT WHAT SITES YOU CAN LOOK AT ON THESE COMPUTERS.

NORMALLY THE SITES THAT THEY ALLOW YOU TO LOOK AT ARE WORK RELATED, OR ABOUT TRAVEL, 'FACEBOOK', AND MANY, MANY OTHERS.

UN-FORTUNATELY MANY PEOPLE ABUSE THE TRUST THAT IS PLACED IN THEM AND TRY TO LOOK AT RESTRICTED SITES. EVEN THOUGH THE COMPUTERS MAY BE MONITORED AND IT MAY MEAN THE 'LOSS' OF COMPUTERS FOR EVERYONE'S USE.

IF USING A COMPUTER, DON'T ABUSE THE PRIVILEGE.

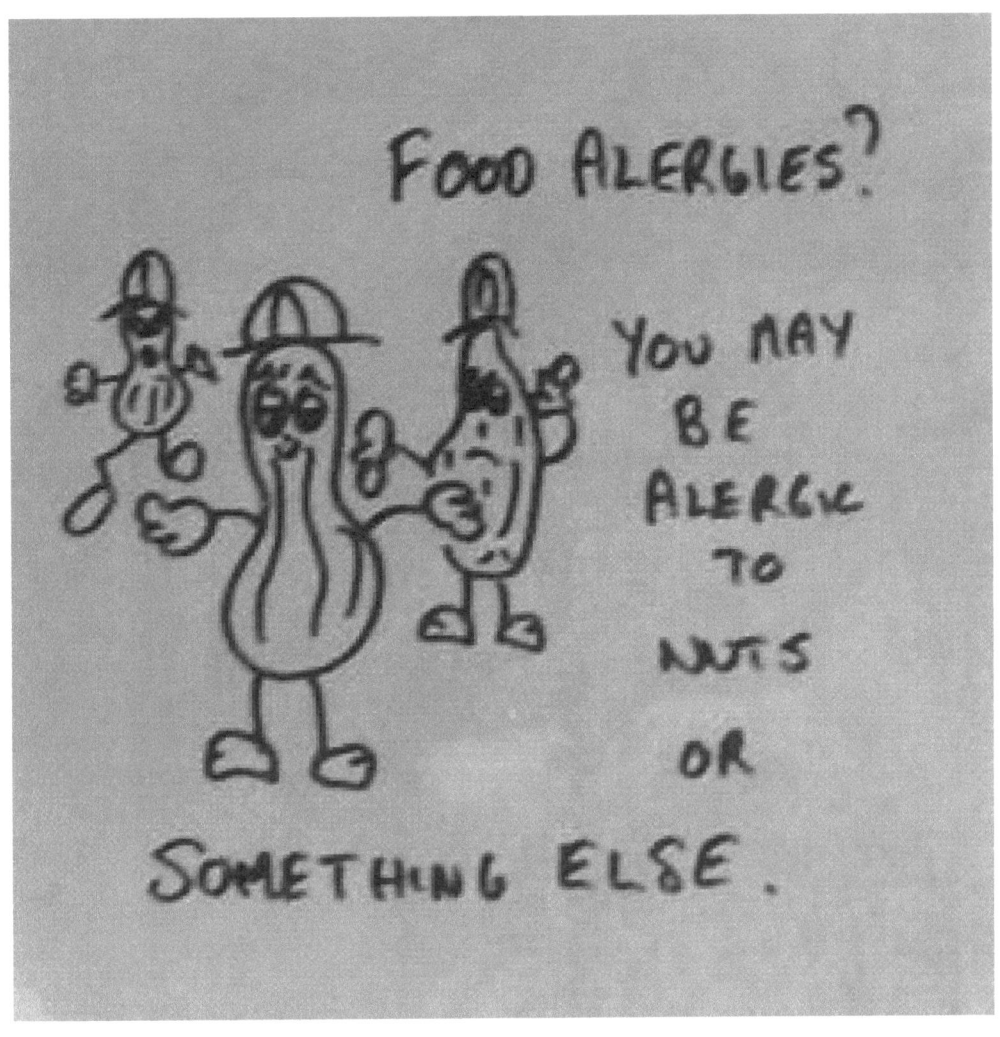

A LOT OF PEOPLE THESE DAYS ARE ALLERGIC TO DIFFERENT CHEMICALS, SOME OF WHICH MAY BE CONTAINED IN THE FOOD THAT WE EAT.

IF YOU ARE WORKING ON A MINE SITE OR ANY OTHER PLACE YOU SHOULD ASK WHAT IS CONTAINED IN THE FOOD.

ESPECIALLY IF YOU ARE ALLERGIC TO SOMETHING LIKE NUTS OR CERTAIN FOOD ADDITIVES

MOST PLACES WILL BE HAPPY TO LET YOU KNOW WHAT THE FOOD CONTAINS. ALSO, IF YOU DO HAVE A REACTION TO SOME FOOD ITEM, FIND OUT WHAT IT CONTAINED AND LET YOUR DOCTOR OR OH & S DEPARTMENT KNOW.

IT'S BETTER TO KNOW WHAT YOU ARE EATING WHEN YOU'RE ALLERGIC TO SOMETHING.

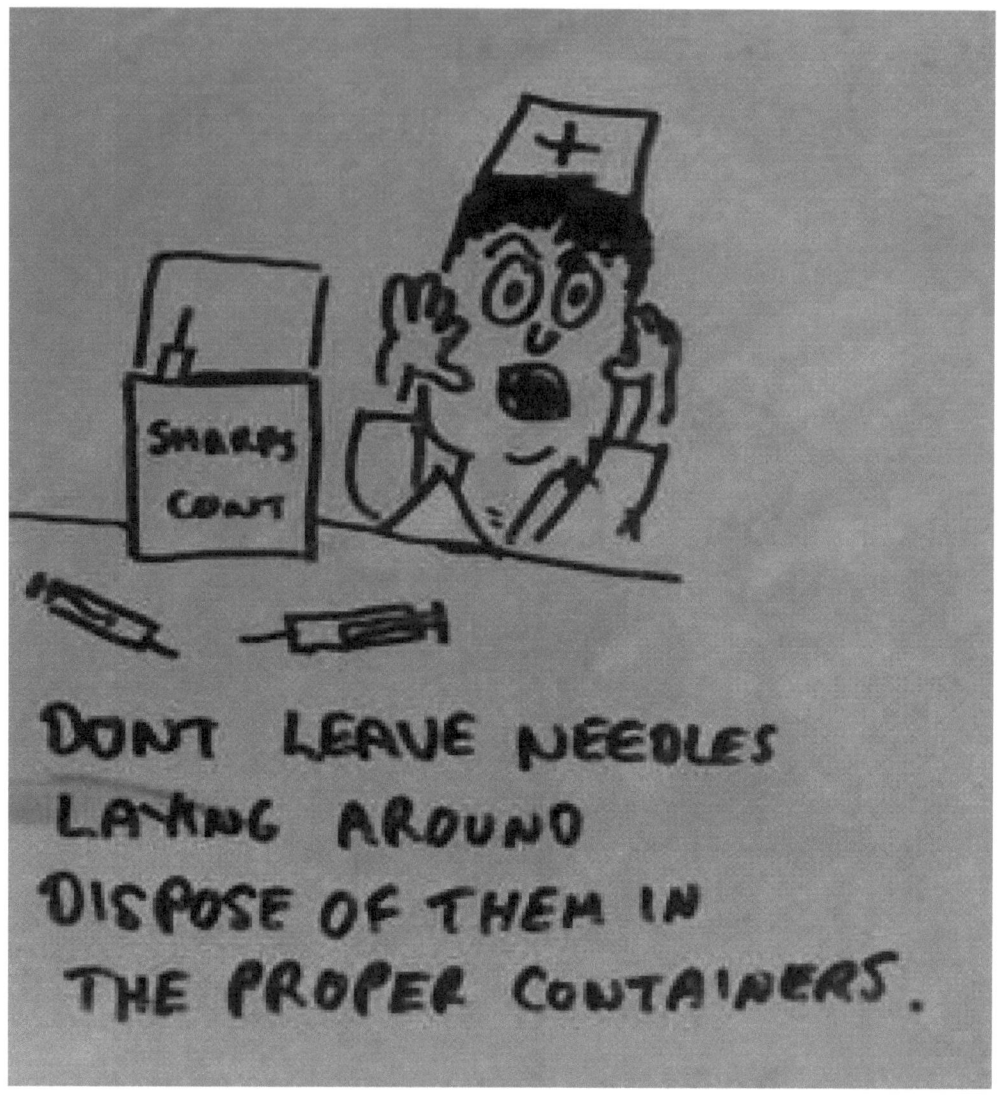

MANY WORK PLACES HAVE 'SHARPS CONTAINERS' IN WHICH NEEDLES CAN BE PLACED AFTER USE.

NORMALLY IT IS THE DOCTOR OR MEDIC THAT USES SUCH ITEMS, BUT SOME PEOPLE WHO HAVE MEDICAL CONDITIONS MAY NEED TO SELF MEDICATE AND THUS NEED SOME TYPE OF CONTAINER TO PUT THE USED SYRINGES IN.

PEOPLE SOMETIMES FORGET TO DO THIS AND CAN DISCARD THEM IN A PUBLIC OR EASILY ACCESSIBLE PLACE.

SO, IF YOU DO SELF MEDICATE OR USE SYRINGES, THINK OF OTHERS AND KEEPTHEM IN A SAFE & SECURE PLACE.

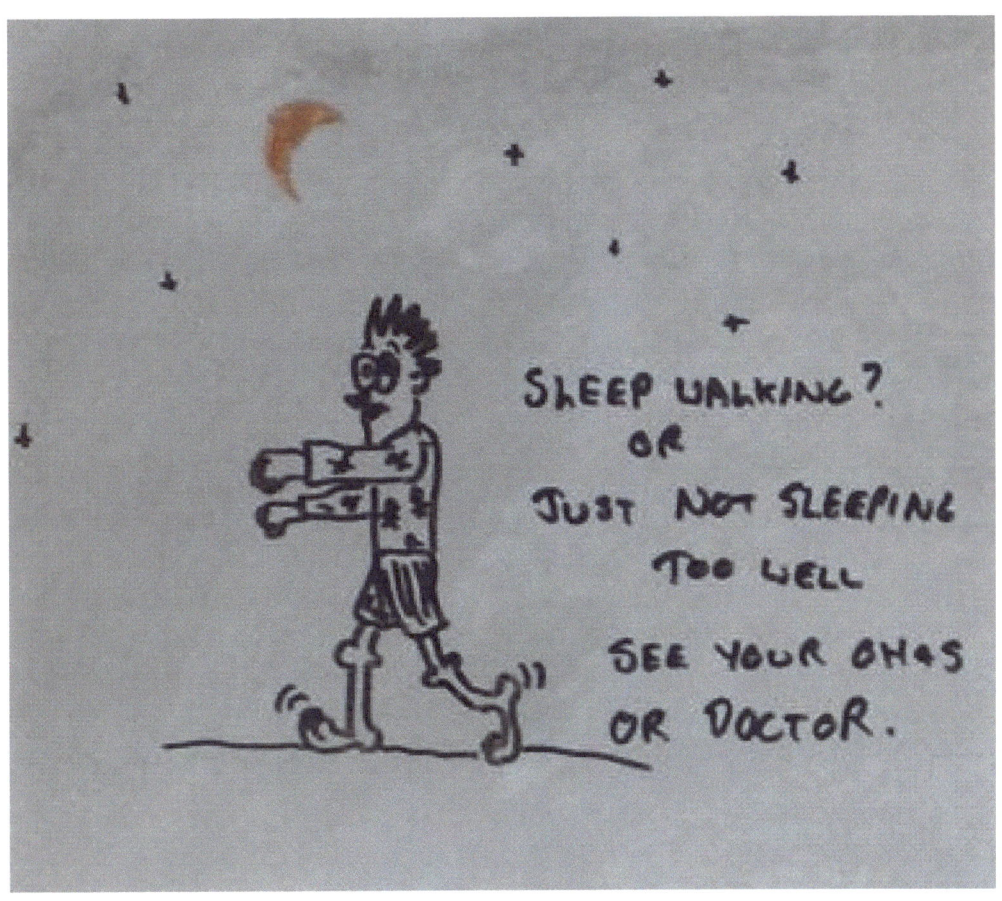

DON'T LAUGH, IT CAN HAPPEN TO ANYONE.

I KNOW THAT I USED TO SLEEP WALK AS A KID AND I HAVE KNOWN SOME ADULTS TO DO THE SELF SAME THING.

IT CAN MEAN THAT YOU ARE NOT GETTING ENOUGH REST AT NIGHT, HAVE SOMETHING ON YOUR MIND, HAVE A BELLY FULL OF FOOD, ARE OVER TIRED, TAKING THE WRONG MEDICATION OR ANY NUMBER OF REASONS.

IF THIS DOES HAPPEN, EITHER ON A MINE SITE, HOME OR ANYWHERE ELSE, YOU SHOULD GO SEE SOME-ONE TO SEE IF THEY CAN HELP YOU.

IF NOT, THEN WHO KNOWS WHAT CAN HAPPEN.

YOU MAY WALK INTO THINGS, INTO TRAFFIC, GET VIOLENT IF WOKEN UP AND NO-ONE WANTS ANY OF THAT TO HAPPEN.

SO SLEEP TIGHT AND JUST ENJOY THE NIGHT…ZZZZZZZZZZZZZZZZZZZZ

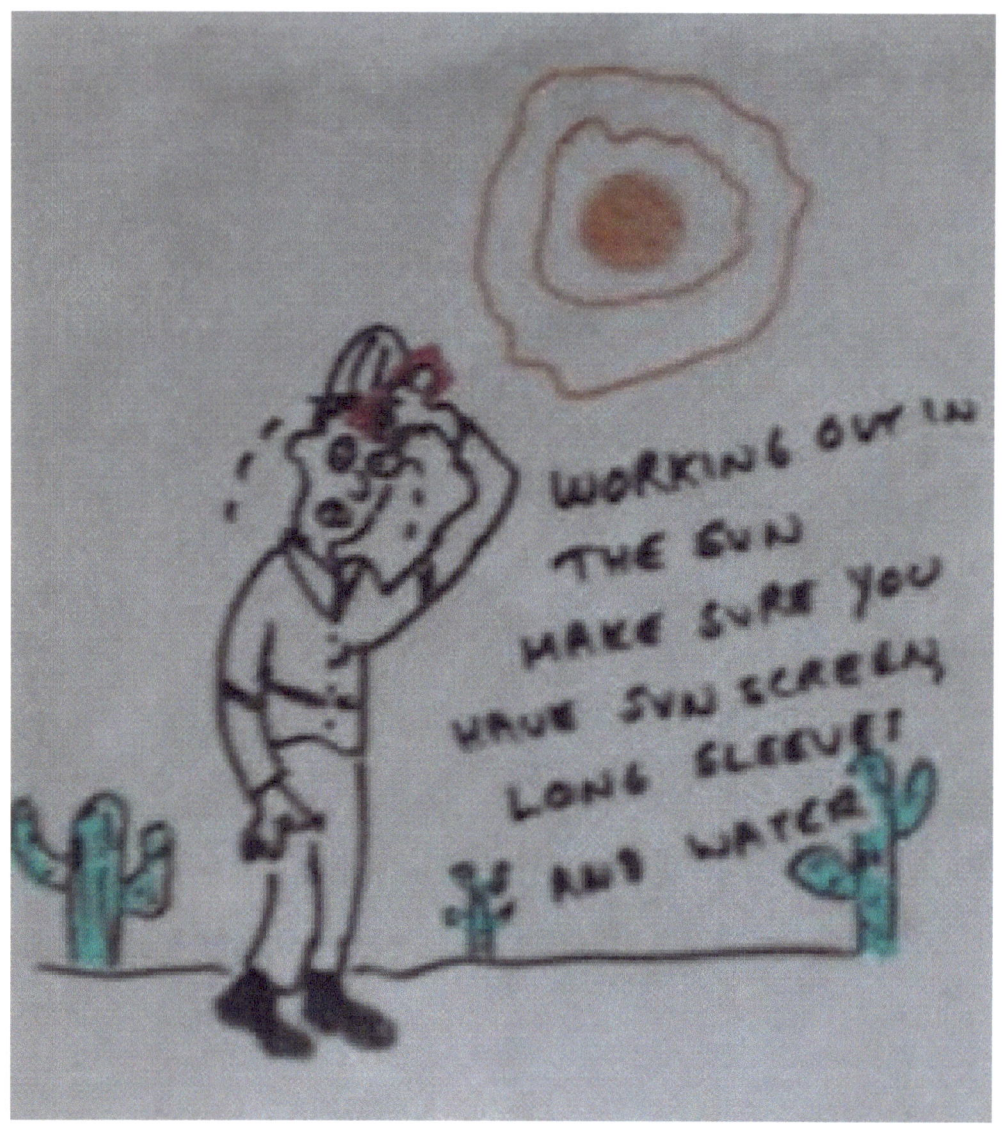

WHEN YOU WORK IN HOT, HUMID OR ARID CONDITIONS YOU HAVE TO REMEMBER SOME BASIC RULES.

ALWAYS WEAR LONG SLEEVES FOR PROTECTION FROM THE SUN AND TO GIVE SOME SORT OF PROTECTION FOR YOUR ARMS.

MAKE SURE THAT YOU WEAR SUNSCREEN ON ALL AREAS THAT ARE OPEN TO THE SUN.

REMEMBER THE OLD ADAGE "SLIP, SLOP, SLAP"

AND DRINK LOTS OF PROPER FLUIDS TO KEEP HYDRATED.

Progressives

This is where you start with one drawing and the theme runs with the continuity of the different drawings.

In this set, we start with 3d; then the netters (who are spiders); a squadron of flies trying to fly into a spider's web, but are stopped by a line of cones and then finally we have an ice-cream van driving around wondering where they left some ice-cream cones.

So from 1 drawing we now end up with 4 in the series.

It's good for moral and it's also good to get the thought processes working as well as being great fun. Safety also means clearing your head and trying different things so that everyone can come together.

How progressive are you?

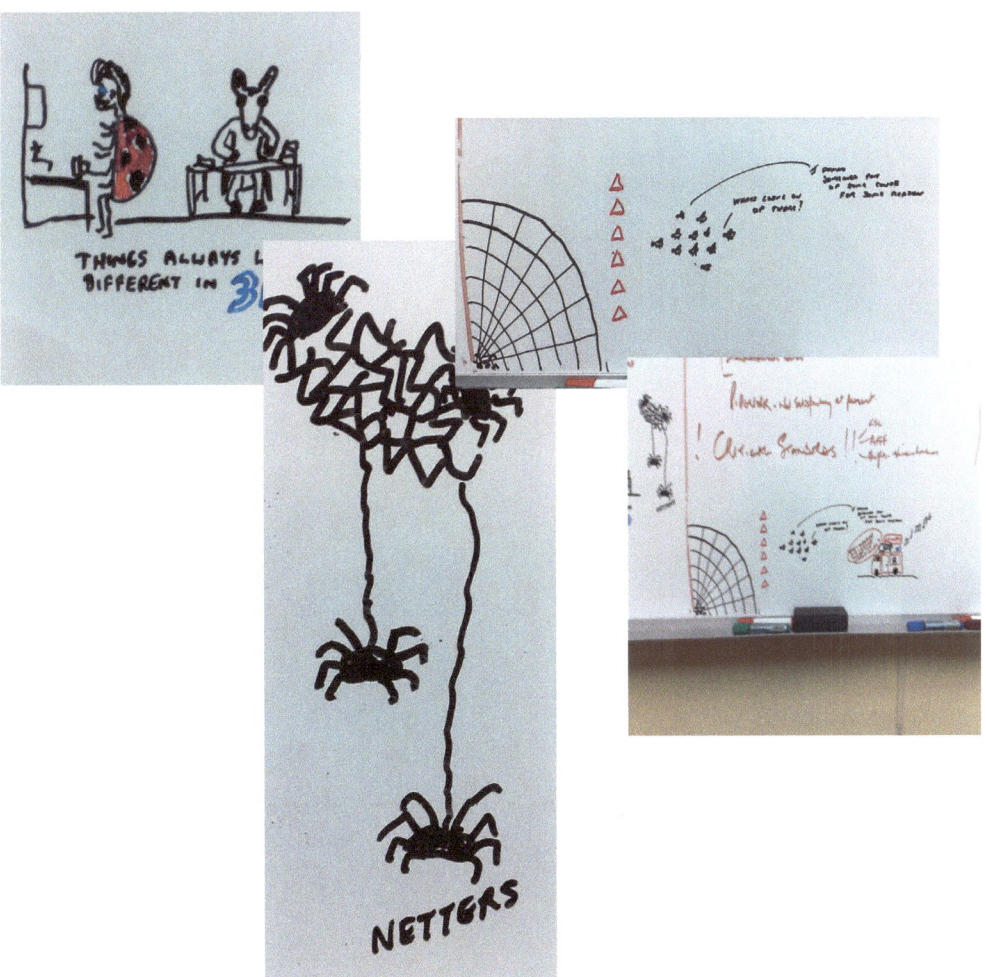

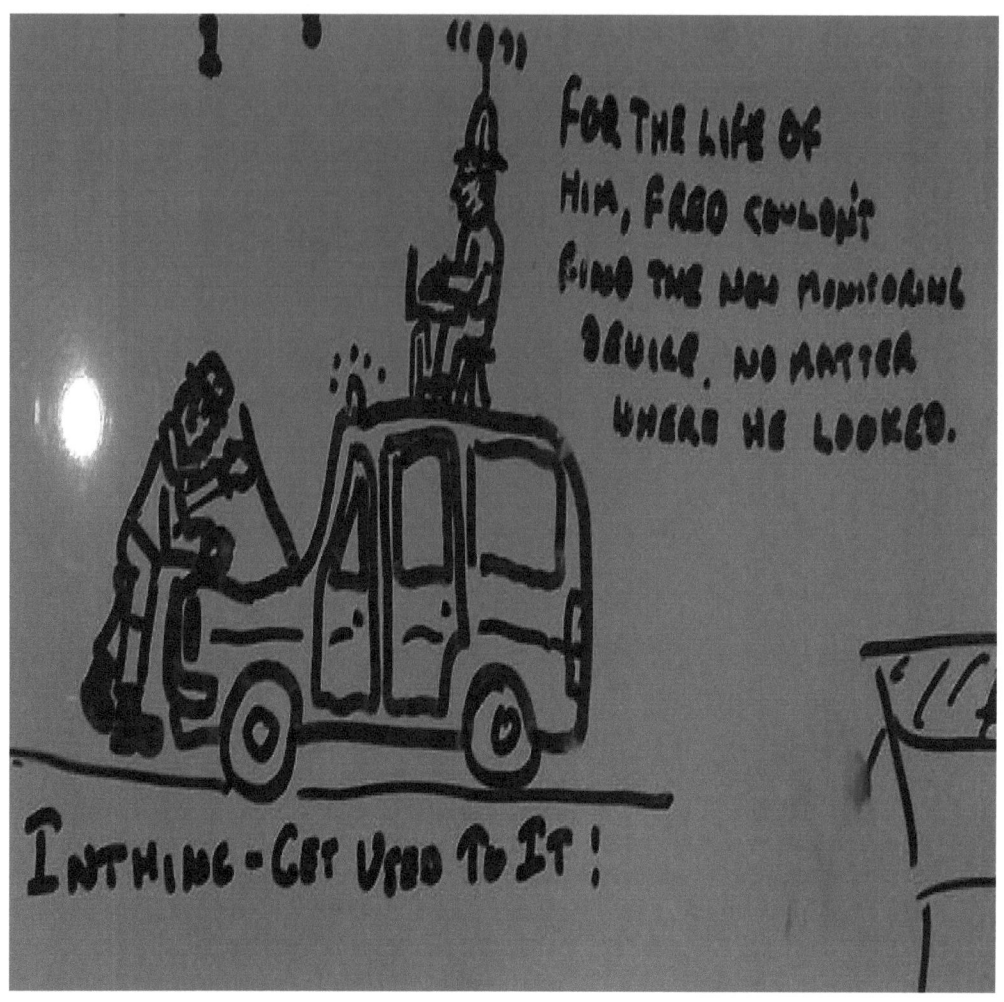

AT THE MINE, THEY HAVE INSTALLED MONITORING DEVICES ON VEHICLES, CALLED 'INTHINC'.

BY INSTALLING THESE DEVICES, IT'S NOT THE OLD ADAGE OF "BIG BROTHER IS WATCHING YOU", BUT A WAY OF IMPROVING DRIVER AWARENESS & LEARNING, PRO-ACTIVE MAINTENANCE BY SAFER DRIVING TECHNIQUES AND ALSO, SO THE COMPANY CAN LEARN TO IMPROVE THEIR DELIVERY PROCEDURES.

IT MAKES ME THINK THAT THIS SYSTEM WOULD ALSO BE ADVANTAGESS FOR MANY OTHER MOTORISTS AROUND THE WORLD TO HELP KEEP THE ROADS A SAFER & BETTER PLACE.

DRIVE SAFE - DRIVE WELL - DRIVE TO SURVIVE

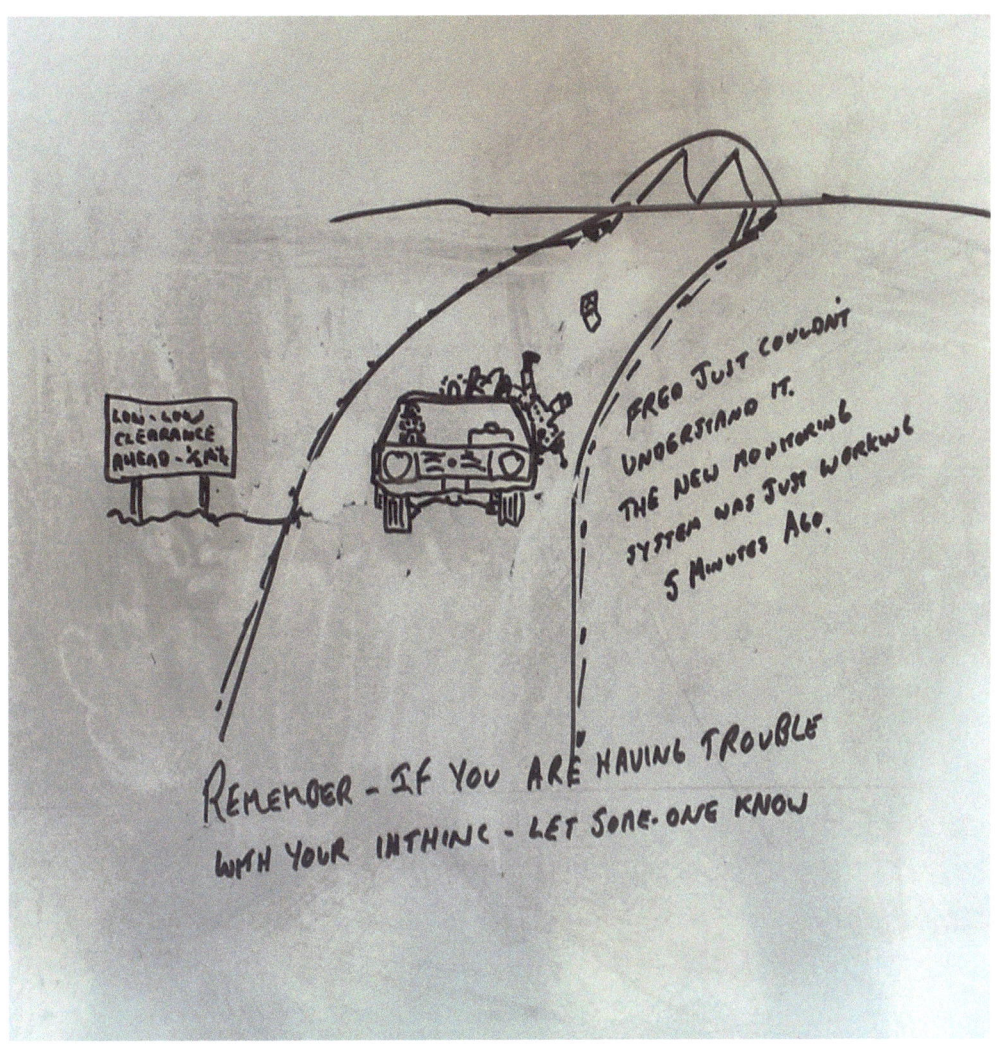

IF YOUR 'INTHINC' SYSTEM FAILS OR IF ANYTHING ELSE BREAKS DOWN, WE NEED TO GET IT FIXED AND BACK UP AND RUNNING.

ALL TOO OFTEN IT IS SO EASY TO LEAVE IT AND LET SOME-ONE ELSE GET IT DONE.

PEOPLE HAVE TO START TO TAKE CARE AND RESPONSIBILITY FOR THEIR ACTIONS AND THE SAFETY OF OTHERS.

BROKEN THINGS SHOULD EITHER BE REPLACED OR REPAIRED.

DON'T BE LEFT OUT IN THE COLD BECAUSE OF SOME-ONE ELSE'S INACTIVITY.

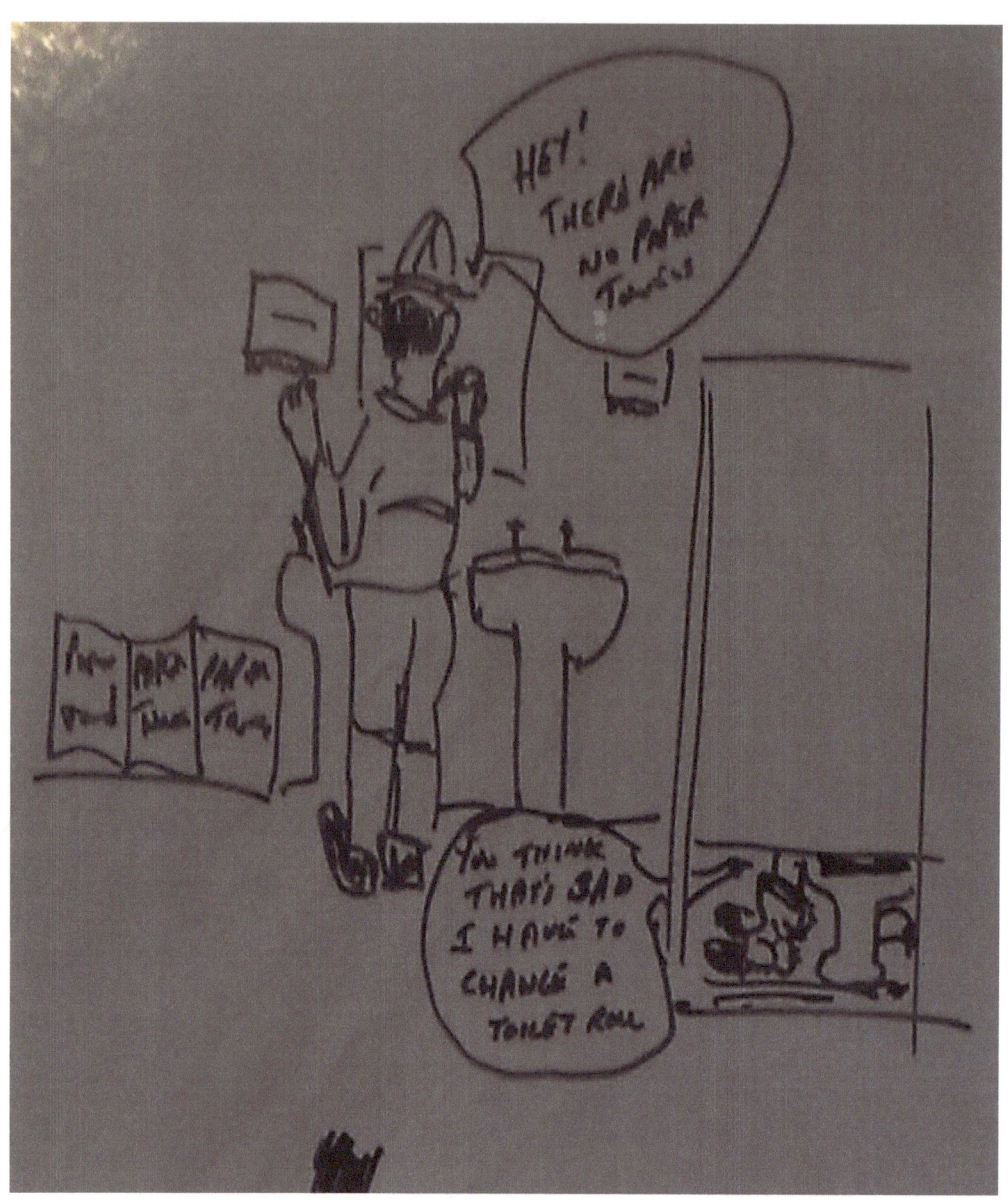

SOMETIMES YOU WOULD THINK THAT THE MOST BASIC OF CONCEPT 'OF DOING SOMETHING FOR YOURSELF' WOULD BE SO EASY.

WRONG!

ONCE AN ITEM HAS BEEN FINISHED, CHANGE IT OUT FOR A NEWER ONE, BECAUSE ANOTHER PERSON MAY WANT TO USE IT AFTER YOU.

BE RESPONSIBLE!

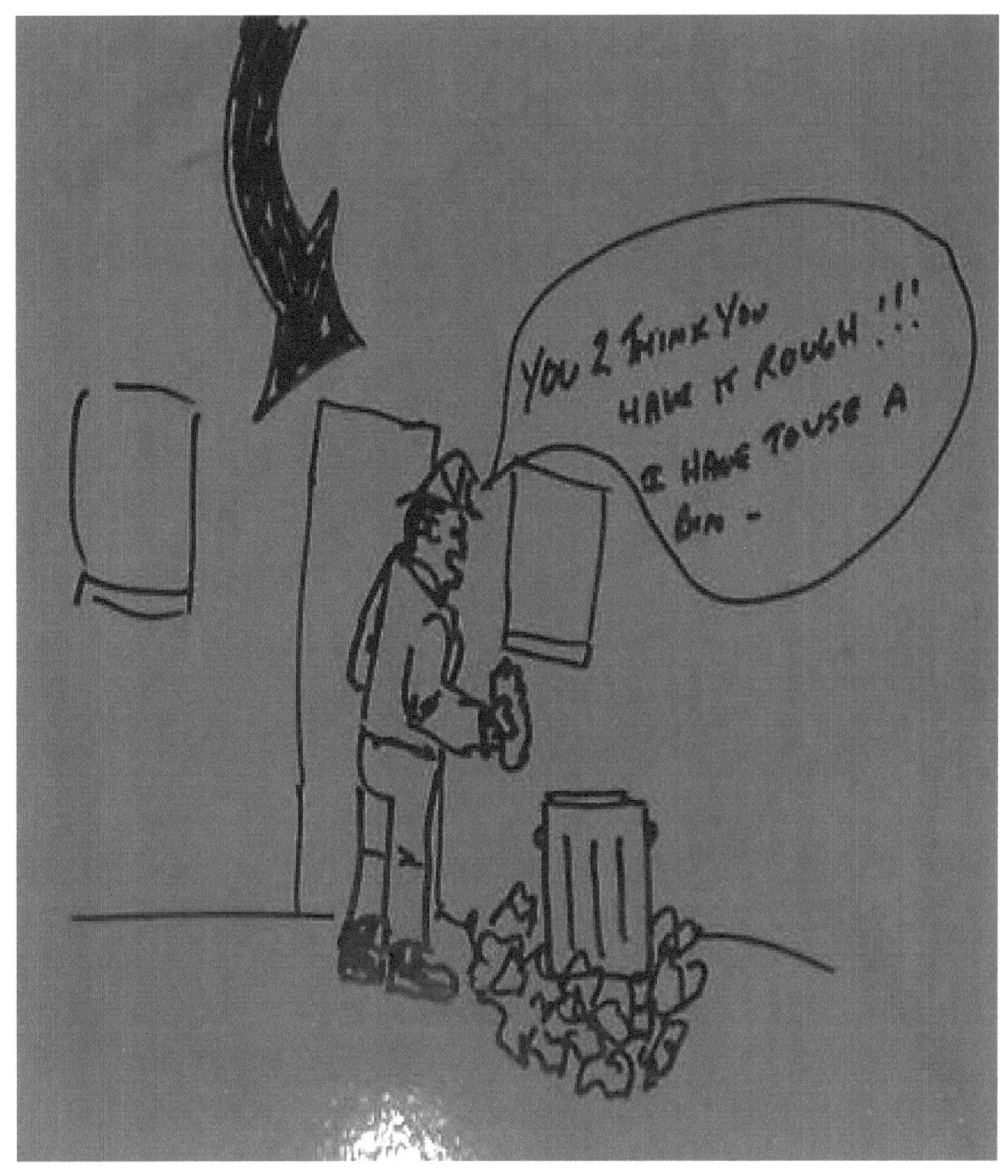

NEED I SAY IT?

RUBBISH - RUBBISH - RUBBISH

IT IS TRULY AMAZING HOW PEOPLE CAN BE ONLY A FEW FEET AWAY FROM A BIN AND FAIL TO USE IT.

THEY CAN EVEN TRY TO THROW IT INTO THE BIN, MISS AND THEN JUST WALK AWAY LEAVING IT ON THE GROUND.

WE NEED TO RESPECT WHERE WE WORK, LIVE AND THOSE THAT HAVE TO PUT UP WITH THIS KIND OF BEHAVIOUR.

WILL OTHERS DRAW?

You might say "this is the million dollar question"

When I first started my drawings, I did not expect the guys down at

Innotech site services to do some for me in return and I believe that they did not expect me to draw a picture of myself in the first place.

In a way I believe that it has to do with the mentality of those involved.

"Should I?"

"What if some-one catches me and I'm embarrassed?"

"What if they are no good?…I went to uni"

In one of the drawings that I had over in the mining offices, I had spots which were numbered, but had left blank, hoping that they may draw themselves in the empty spaces.

But alas, I was disappointed.

No such luck.

So instead of letting the thought get to me, I continued on drawing.

Although it is hard sometimes to know if they are appreciated or not, you just have to 'wing' it.

I'm sure that if they were upset that a cleaner or some-one else who was 'not of their fraternity' had done such work, they would have let   me know.

Maybe they are just scared because they feel that the scope of such work is out of their job description.

But…don't worry, because it will happen one day.

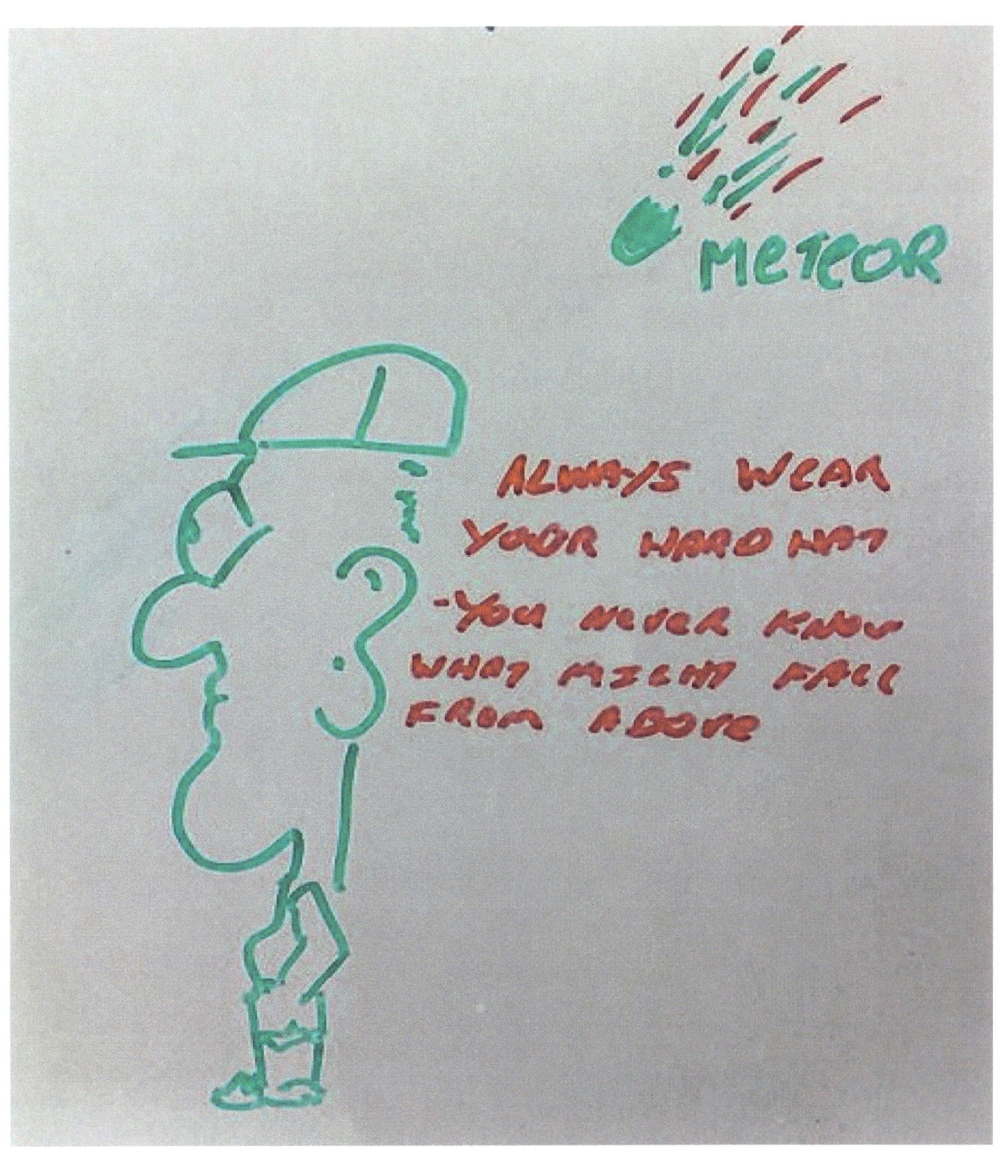

((DRAWN BY ERIK STOKES)

HARD HATS ARE PART OF SOME WORK PLACE PPE (PERSONAL PROTECTION EQUIPMENT).

IF YOU WALK UNDER STRUCTURES OR ARE OUT IN THE OPEN ON MINING SITES OR CONSTRUCTION SITES, ETC, IT MAKES COMMON SENSE TO PROTECT YOUR MOST VALUABLE ASSET.

YOUR HEAD.

THINK SMART - THINK SAFE - PROTECT YOUR ASSETS

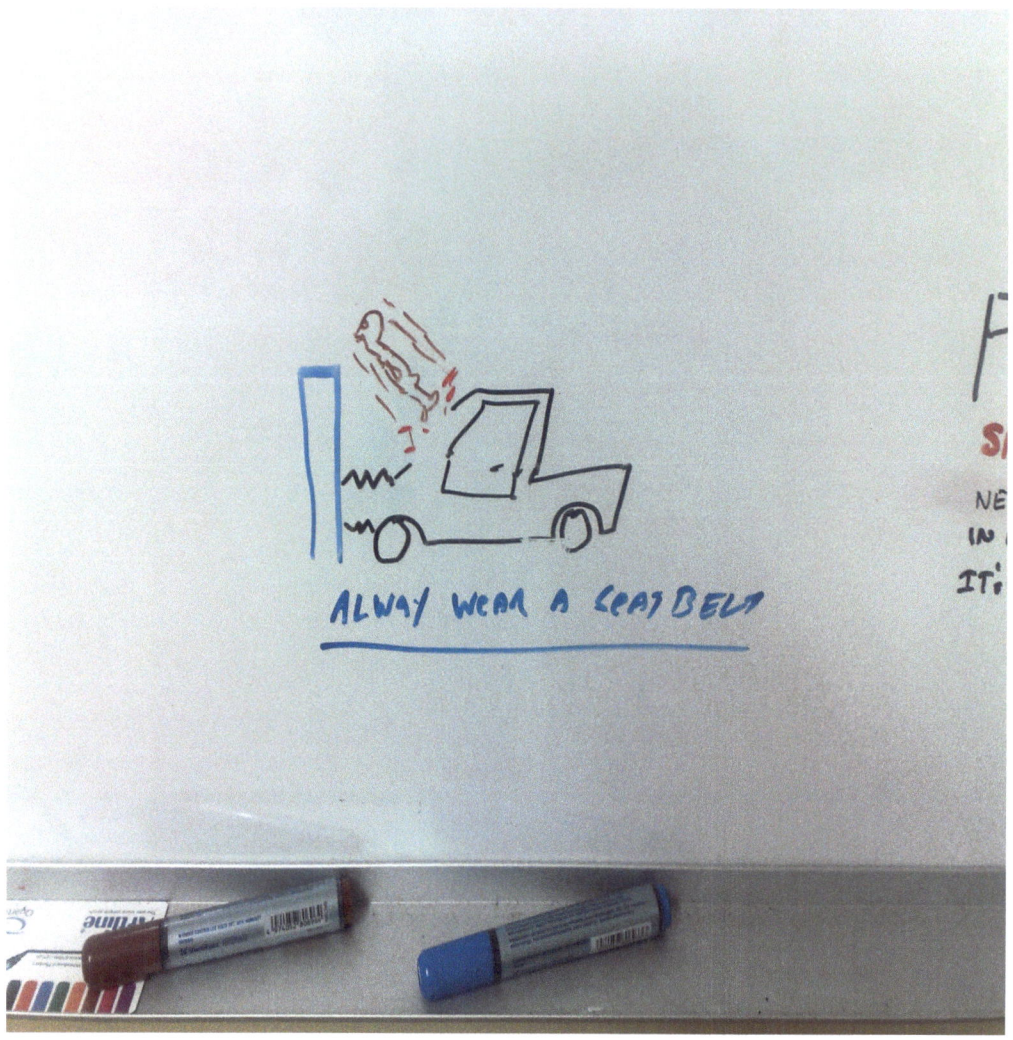

((DRAWN BY ERIK STOKES)

SEATBELTS, CLICK!

IN AUSTRALIA, IT IS COMPULSORY TO WEAR YOUR SEATBELT WHEN YOU ARE TRAVELLING IN A CAR OR TRUCK. IT DOES NOT MATTER IF YOU ARE THE DRIVER OR THE PASSENGER.

YOU STILL HAVE TO WEAR ONE.

WHY? BECAUSE STATISTICS HAVE SHOWN THAT IF YOU ARE WEARING A SEATBELT IN AN ACCIDENT, YOUR CHANCES OF SURVIVING A CRASH ARE VERY GOOD.

SEE; THERE IS AN UPSIDE.!

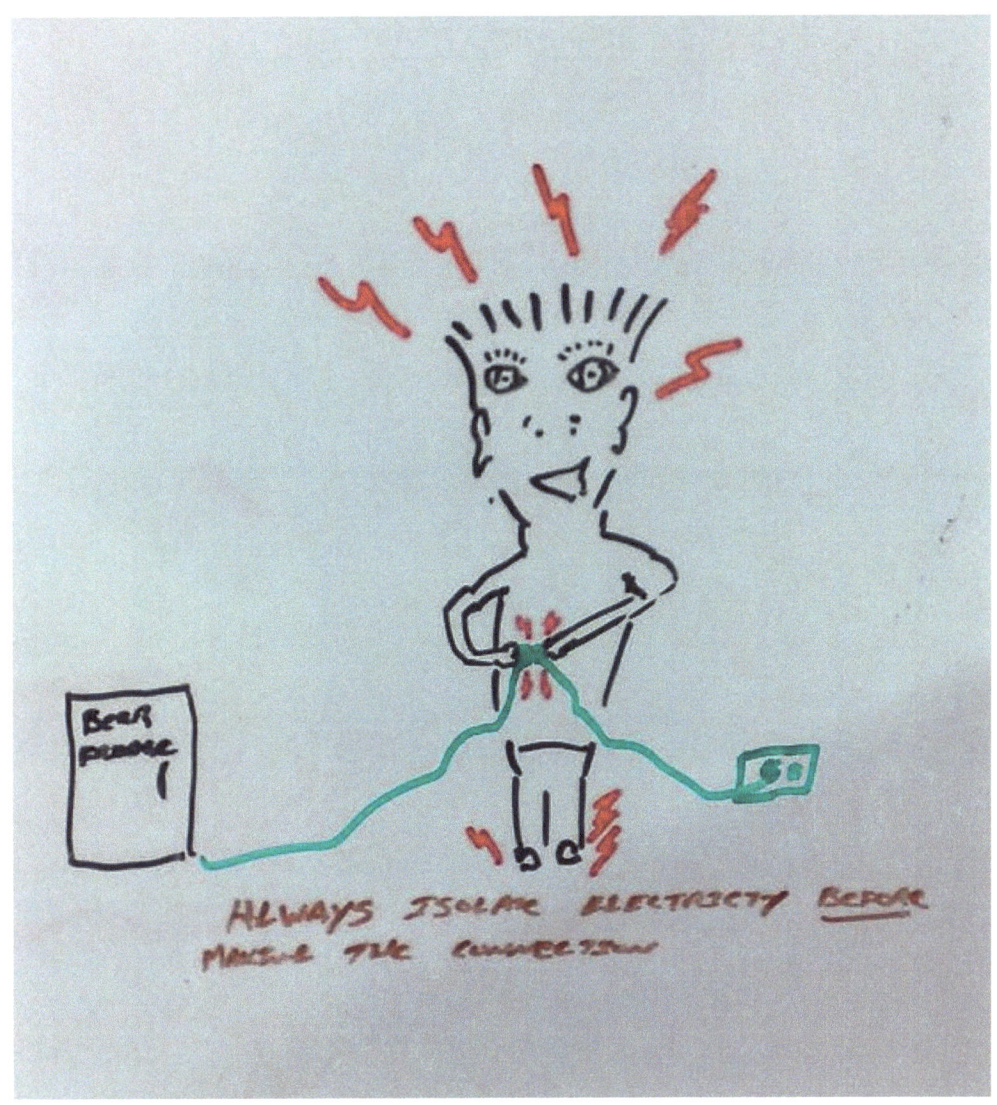

((DRAWN BY ERIK STOKES)

ELECTRICITY KILLS, SINGES, BURNS AND ALL THE ASSOCIATED STUFF.

ONE OF THE MOST BASIC RULES THAT WE LEARN FROM BEING CHILDREN, IS TO SWITCH OFF THE POWER SWITCH IF WE ARE CONNECTING ELECTRICAL EQUIPMENT AND THEN ONCE IT IS PLUGGED IN, YOU CAN TURN IT ON AGAIN.

EVEN WITH THIS HEAD START IN COMMON SENSE, PEOPLE ARE STILL GETTING ELECTROCUTED BECAUSE THEY FORGOT TO ISOLATE THE POWER.

WHY DO WE FORGET, ELECTRICITY CAN KILL?

SAYINGS & WORDS IN WORKING

If you cannot draw, too well, then do not worry. You may have what is called "the gift of the gab."

You may be able to string words together to make sense of the insensible, or at least, enable those who matter the most, can at least understand the thought behind the words.

No amount of words will replace good old natural 'know how', but if it saves one life or makes some-one stop doing a silly act.

Then it is all worth it!

THE CEMETARIES ARE
FULL OF PEOPLE
WHO THOUGHT THAT
IT WAS SAFE.

- STAY ALIVE - BE SAFE

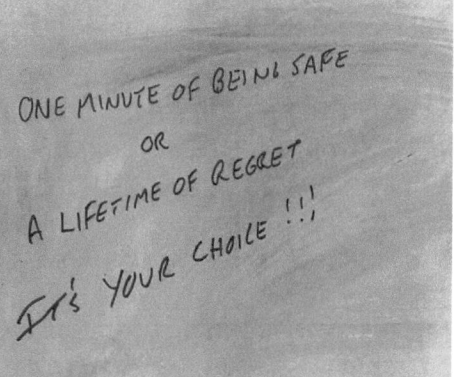

ONE MINUTE OF BEING SAFE
OR
A LIFETIME OF REGRET
IT'S YOUR CHOICE !!!

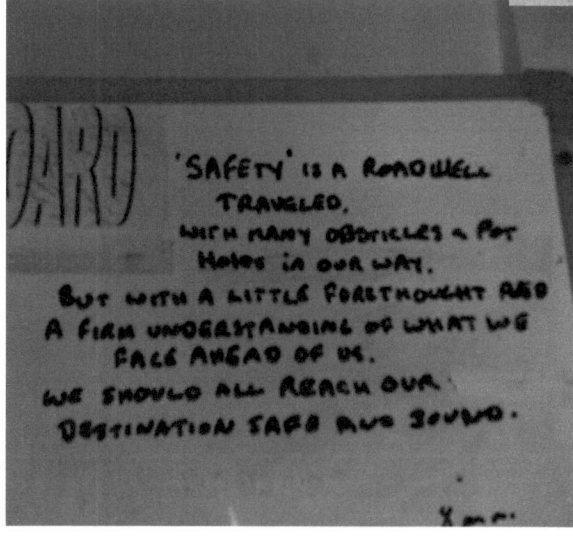

'SAFETY' IS A ROAD WELL
TRAVELED,
WITH MANY OBSTACLES & POT
HOLES IN OUR WAY.
BUT WITH A LITTLE FORETHOUGHT AND
A FIRM UNDERSTANDING OF WHAT WE
FACE AHEAD OF US.
WE SHOULD ALL REACH OUR
DESTINATION SAFE AND SOUND.

Being safe is a way to share with everyone. Being un-safe is just a way of showing how greedy you really are.

Be skilled not killed

Don't let some-one you know stop you from going home tonight.
Work safe

Hard hat or just a hard head? Wear ya helmut.

WORK COMPETITIONS & POSSIBLE INCENTIVE PROGRAMS FOR ALL

We need to look at also the use of competitions and incentives to keep both staff and contractors on track with their safety, because after a while they will lose sight of the goals that you wish them to achieve.

With this in mind, I have included an idea here for everyone to have a look at and maybe try out.

Who knows, it may even catch on and become part of any companies safety regime on a regular basis.

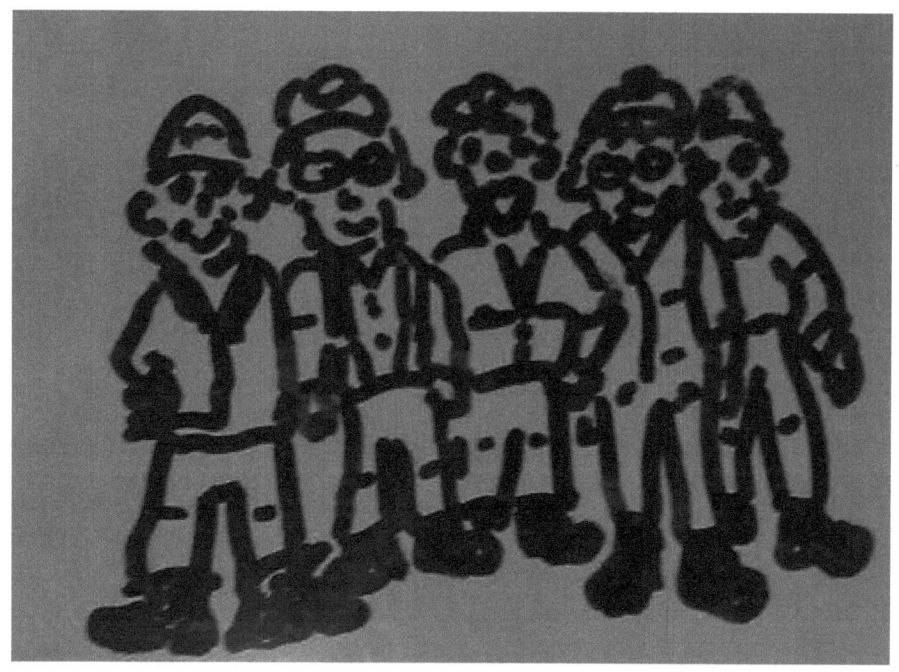

ISN'T IT TIME? INCENTIVE IDEA

I modeled this one after one of the cartoons that I had done and I thought what a great name for a safety competition.

What we would do is all departments & sections and then all the different crews within those (i.e. crew a, crew b etc.) would all be working on the 'buddy' system. That is, they would each have to look out for each other to make sure that no accidents, near misses, transgressions occurred within a specific time frame; because if any of these happened they would lose points as a group.

To gain points they could 'pick up' other problems from other groups. I know this may lead to 'un-necessary' reports, but those should be discouraged and maybe even penalized if too frequent.

If the crews or the departments have varying numbers of people within them, then you would use a ratio system to bring all the different areas onto an equal footing.

Ideally this competition would run for approximately for 3 months, because as with any work competition or incentive program they can run for too long and lose impetuous and then the people involved will lose sight of what is trying to be achieved.

It could also be beneficial to have monthly spot prizes or incentives for the best group or even the best safety message as drawn on a whiteboard etc., but that would be up to the different companies involved.

The prizes or incentives do not need to be big, but then not too small either (unless you try some novelty prizes for 'fun' value.

With the advent of these monthly prizes and varying the topics/discussions you are keeping everyone's focus and hopefully they do not lose their enthusiasm for the event.

Give it a try - if it works great; if it doesn't, well the only thing lost was 'not trying anything at all'.

VARIATIONS IN THE DRAWINGS & FLASH LIGHT SPOTS

As I have talked about earlier, not all the drawings will be identical when you do multiples of them in different places.

You can add changes, or props as it were to make it more acceptable to the people you wish to reach.

Some may look okay, while others are so-so.

But as with anything in life, you take what you can get, so don't worry, just accept it.

I do and so should you.

One thing I will mention, which you would have seen already. Some of the pictures have 'flash' or 'light spots' in them. This is because I usually take a photo of them with my nokia mobile phone.

I could have edited them out, but I ask myself why?

I don't wish to look like a professional 'air brushed' model, but rather something which is natural and down to earth.

So, if you don't like it or if it upsets you, well that is life.

Being vain is not a necessity, but being yourself is.

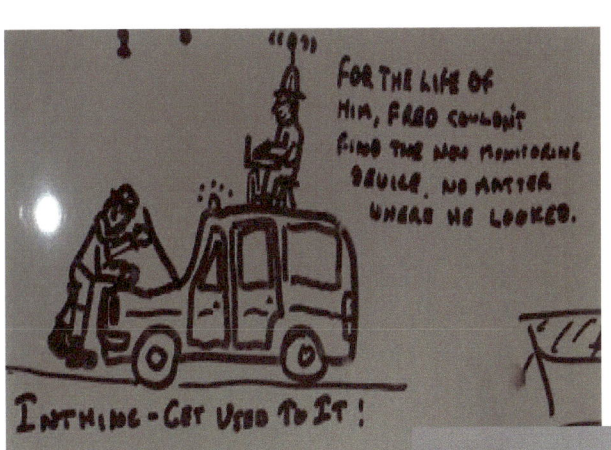
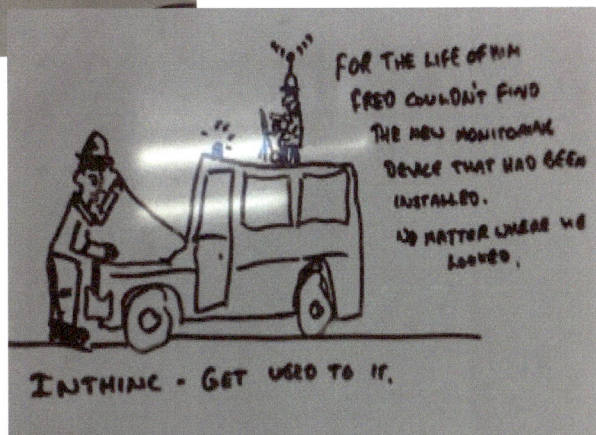
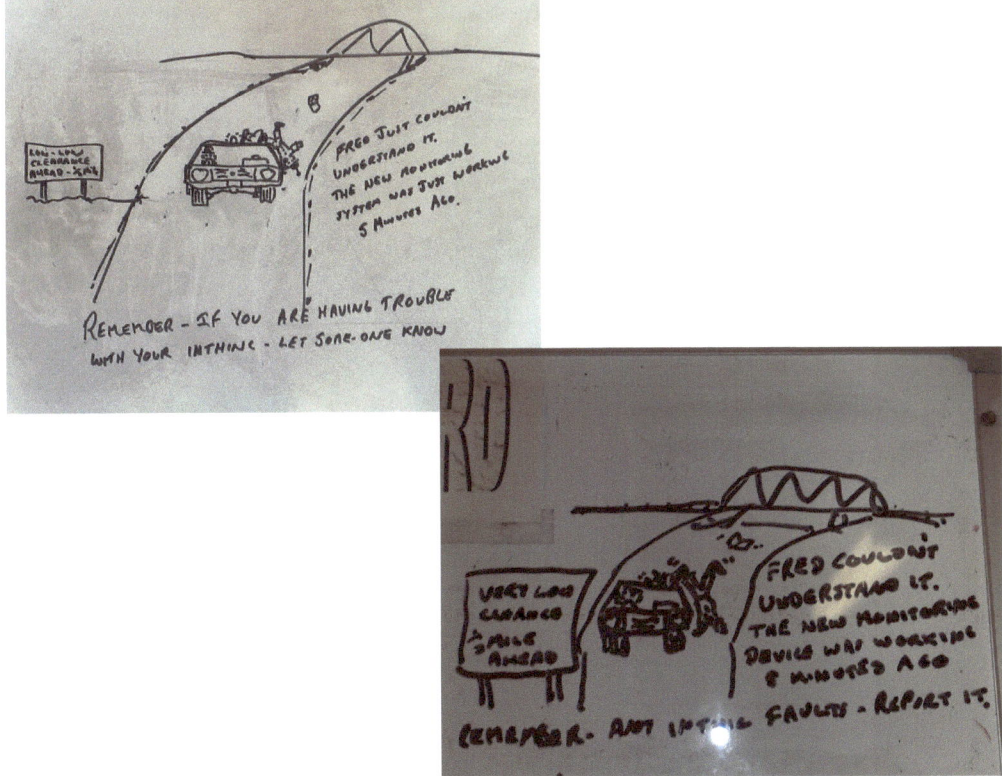

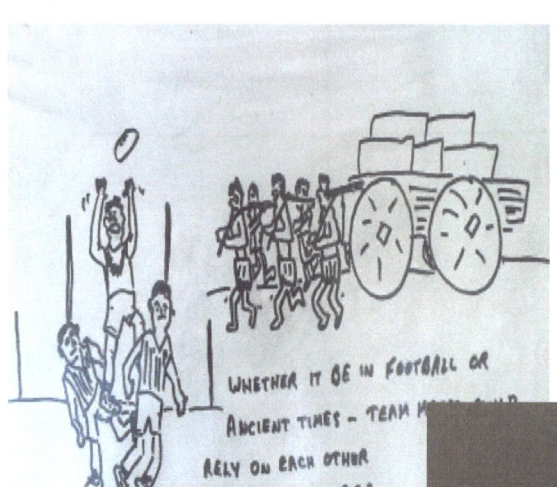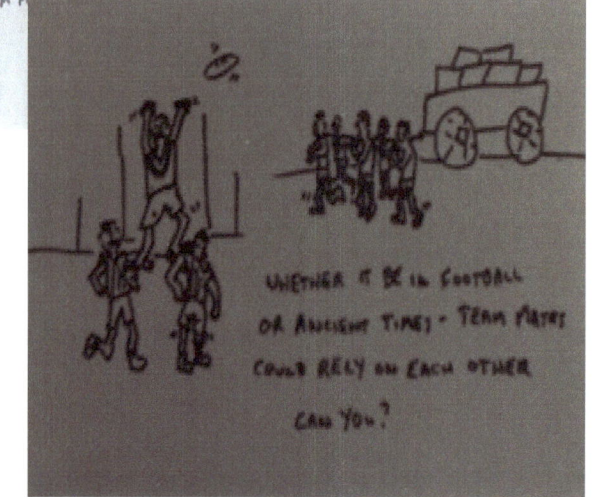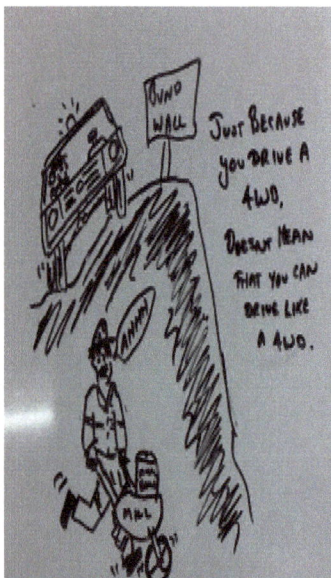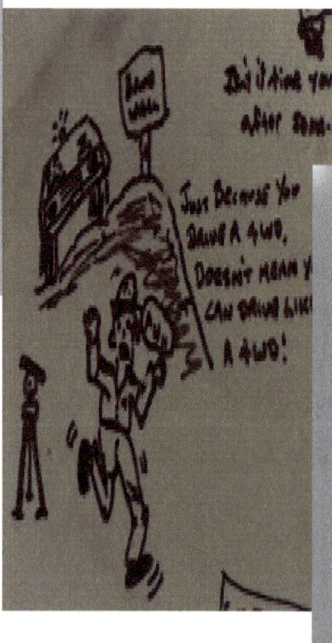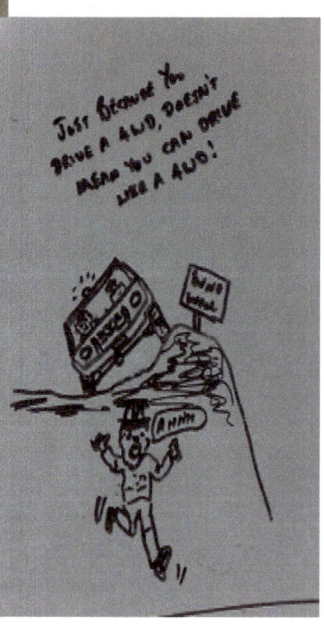

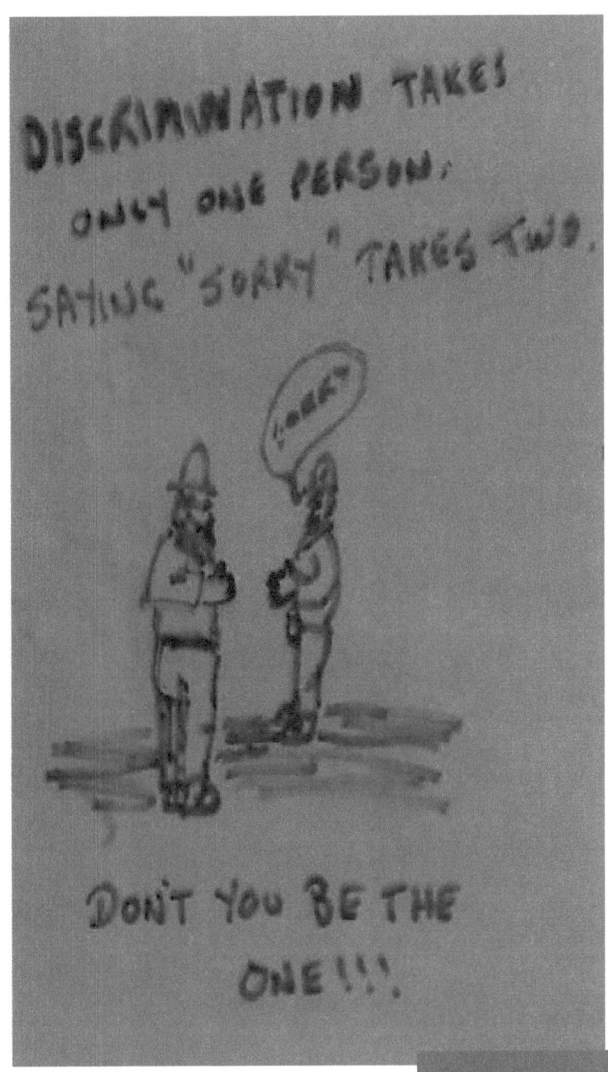

The sayings are different, but they both mean the selfsame thing.

So drawing variations can and will be different.

Especially if you forgot what you wrote in the first place.

but that doesn't matter just as long as it is basically the same.

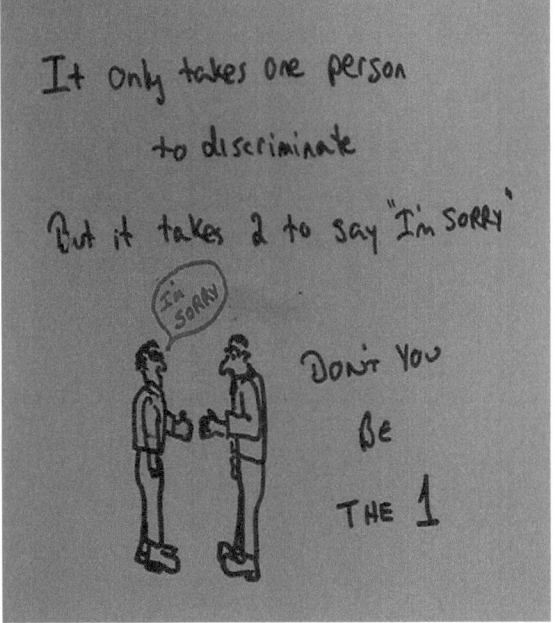

AND FINALLY…BLACKBOARDS & EASELS

If you do not have any access to whiteboards, you can always use blackboards or even those easels, which hold those flip chart paper books.

With whiteboards and the blackboards you can always make changes as you draw, but with the easels you have a greater difficulty in doing that.

The first time I drew on an easel, I found that I did not like the drawing as it was progressing, so I ripped it off and started again. Then I thought to myself, "This will go through heaps of paper if I keep doing this" so I now do the drawings and just hope that they look okay.

If they don't, well, I guess that I and everyone else will have to put up with them as they are.

You can see with this picture, that I have three drawings on the same page.

As I drew them, I kept thinking "will they turn out ok?"

I believe that they did, so I was happy.

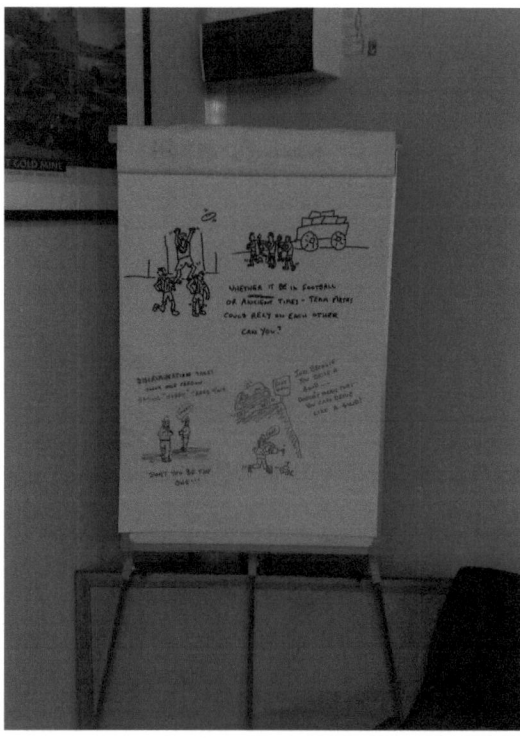

Even if they didn't, it was not worth wasting paper on trying to look perfect.

It's just not worth it.

WHAT THEY "SAY"

FRED

"You might recognize me from the inthinc sketches. Since I started appearing in these I have come to appreciate why we have these systems installed in the vehicles that we drive. I know that my driving has improved and I know that others have as well".

"Now all I need to do is have one installed in my son's car." "So, take care & safe driving."

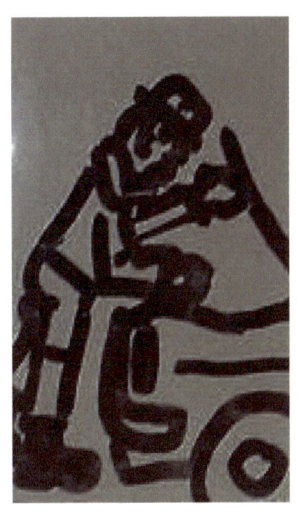

DEATH

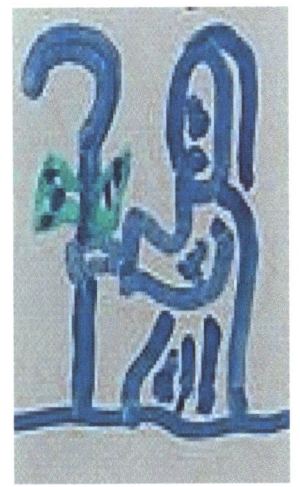

Death talks about the mistake he made by grabbing a 'Sheppard's crook' instead of his 'trademark scythe'. "It was so easy. I didn't realize that using the right tool for the right job was so important. Being in a rush meant that I didn't make my daily quota."

"I'll know better next time."

MUM

"Being some-ones mother is an important job, but they have to leave the nest sometime and then they have to fend for themselves. I just hope that what we teach them as parents stay with them and they don't let anyone down by being unsafe or untidy."

"I love my family and I would miss them terribly if anything happened."

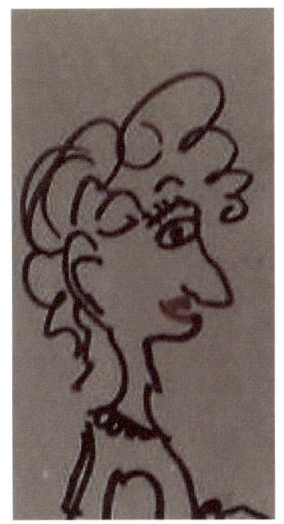

POINTS TO REMEMBER

- When you are doing any drawings or sayings try not to get too personal with them where you can insult a person or persons, because if you do, you run the risk of bordering on discrimination.

- try not to go too close to any other writing on the board which could be important to some-one else. You may accidently rub some of their work off.

- don't be put 'off' if your work gets 'rubbed' off as they may need the whiteboard for something else.

- Safety can include anything from hygiene, type of work, tools

Used, safe procedures, the processors involved, methods etc.

Etc., etc. So anything can and should be included.

- If people start doing their own and they are better than yours,

Don't get displeased, but feel good within yourself that you have started a revolution.

- if you do take up the challenge of becoming a 'whiteboard safetiest' then remember it is open to anyone from managers to line workers; from supervisors to cleaners; from you to me.

Being safe is what counts

GLOSSARY OF TERMS

Safeticality: it is what people who are safe practice.

Whiteboard Safetiest: this is the name given to anyone who draws on whiteboards. Whether it is in cartoons, sayings or any combination of the two.

Inthinc: a monitoring system that can be installed on vehicles to improve the safety techniques of the people driving and in the use of preventable maintenance.

FLRA: (field level risk assessment) this is to assess the risks involved when any task has to be performed. That way you can see what hazards may be associated with the job. It was explicitly introduced and instigated by Barrick

Ppe: personal protection equipment. These are items that a person must wear or have on their person to complete certain work requirements. They are used to protect you from a variety of conditions and hazards.

"CAUSE FOR PAUSE"

A SAFETY FIRST INNITIATIVE

IS IT SAFE TO DO THE JOB?

                                                                 AM I SAFE

ARE MY WORKMATES SAFE?

HAVE I GOT THE RIGHT TOOLS?

AM I USING THE RIGHT PPE?

DO I KNOW THE CORRECT PROCEDURES?

IF YOU ANSWERED 'NO' TO ANY OF THE ABOVE QUESTIONS - THEN 'PAUSE'

AND FIND OUT WHAT YOU DO NEED AND HOW THE JOB SHOULD BE DONE.

DON'T BE THE CAUSE OF A SERIOUS ACCIDENT!!!

THINK SAFE   WORK SAFE   BE SAFE

A NOTE FROM THE AUTHOR

Well, I hope that you enjoyed whiteboard safety and that you found it useful and informative.

Even if you laughed at some of the content, or even frowned because you found it too simplistic, I don't mind at all.

When I started this journey, I was not even sure that I would ever finish it and I believe that I never will. Safety is an ever ongoing concern because tools change, people forget things and become too complacent, machinery is superseded and replaced; work procedures change. Any number of things can change within a workplace, school, home or even when you are out in a public place.

Whiteboard Safety can be used by anyone, you don't need to be a rocket scientist to draw or work out what is safe and what isn't.

All too often we take shortcuts, knowing full well that it is unsafe to do so. Everybody is guilty of it, myself included.

We know that in all probability an accident will not happen, but what do we do if it does? It may not be ourselves that get hurt or even killed, but usually it is someone we know and maybe even care about.

So take the time out to know what you need so that you can complete the job safely.

Take the time out to see if there are any problems that may happen if something
NOTES

Take the time out, so that when you go home at night, you can take the time out to be yourself and to be with your family and friends.

The good thing about Whiteboard Safety is that it can be tailor made to fit any work place, school, learning, home environment.

You're never too young or old to learn about safety.

TAKE CARE AND STAY SAFE

NOTES

NOTES

NOTES

www.ingramcontent.com/pod-product-compliance
Lightning Source LLC
Chambersburg PA
CBHW041512220426
43661CB00047B/1537